Hospital Cost Containment Programs

A Policy Analysis

Hospital Cost Containment Programs

A Policy Analysis

Edward F.X. Hughes, M.D., M.P.H.
David P. Baron, D.B.A.
David A. Dittman, Ph.D.
Bernard S. Friedman, Ph.D.
Beaufort B. Longest, Jr., Ph.D.
Mark V. Pauly, Ph.D.
Kenneth R. Smith, Ph.D.

Center for Health Services and Policy Research
Northwestern University
Evanston, Illinois

Ballinger Publishing Company • Cambridge, Massachusetts
A Subsidiary of Harper & Row, Publishers, Inc.

This book is printed on recycled paper.

International Standard Book Number: 0–88410–705–1

Library of Congress Catalog Card Number: 78–13793

Printed in the United States of America

Library of Congress Cataloging in Publication Data

Main entry under title:

Hospital cost containment programs.

   Includes bibliographical references.   1. Hospitals—United States—Cost control.   2. Hospitals—United States—Cost of operation.
3. Hospitals—United States—Rates.   4. Hospitals—Rates—Law and legislation—United States.
I.   Hughes, Edward F. X.
RA981.A2H575   658.1'552   78–13793
ISBN 0–88410–705–1

Contents

Appendixes

✳

List of Tables

List of Figures

※

Acknowledgments

This book was originally prepared as a component of the
application of the Center for Health Services and Policy
Research of Northwestern University in the national competition for a National Health Services Policy Analysis Center submitted to the National Center for Health Services Research on July 1,
1977. The original manuscript analysed the administration's proposal
for Hospital Cost Containment (HR 6575) and the Talmadge proposal (S 1470). The manuscript has been substantially revised and expanded to include an analysis of the expanded Talmadge principles
of late 1977 as well as of the Rogers and Rostenkowski proposals of
1978, especially as the latter relates to the "Voluntary Effort."

The authors are indebted to many individuals for help in the com-
pletion of this work. We are especially grateful to Martin Drebin,
David Everhart, Earle Frederick, Paul Ginsburg, James Sammons,
M.D., and David Shenker for their helpful comments. We are also
grateful to Judith Hicks, Susan Slotter, Cindy Schweich, Sarah Bates,
Charlotte Bailey, Penelope Kingman, and Carrie Duncan for their
help in the preparation of the manuscript. We are indebted to Mr.
Tryfon Beazoglou for his untiring work and insightful comments.

The authors are also grateful to the members of the Center for
Health Services and Policy Research who served so dutifully on both
the Program Development Committee and the Production Unit during the preparation of our Policy Analysis Center proposal. It was
through their work that we were able to undertake and complete this

book. Among the authors, I would like to thank Kenneth Smith and especially Mark Pauly for their help in the revision.

Edward F.X. Hughes, M.D. M.P.H.

May 1978
Evanston, Illinois

Part I

Executive Summary
and Recommendations

Chapter 1

Introduction

The escalation of the cost of medical care has become a matter of substantial national concern—a concern that manifests itself on two levels. On the one hand, there is concern about the magnitude of the problem. As a percentage of the gross national product, health care expenditures have risen from 5.2 percent in FY 1960 to 8.8 percent in FY 1977. On the other hand, there is concern about the complexity of the problem. The underlying causes of the cost inflation are a set of institutional arrangements that insulate providers and consumers from market incentives. These arrangements can be briefly summarized as follows:

1. The dominant role of insurance has led to a situation in which, once a health problem occurs, the consumer generally lacks direct financial responsibility for his own care; thus, excess utilization can result.
2. The cost-based retrospective reimbursement system has led to a situation in which there are limited incentives for assuring that the appropriate type and intensity of care is provided at a reasonable cost.
3. The traditional inability and/or unwillingness of consumers, providers, and policymakers to address the cost-quality tradeoff has resulted in a situation in which providers strive for improvements in the quality of care almost without regard to cost. The result is a tendency to adopt technological innovations whose ultimate impact on the quality of care is unevaluated and possibly small.

4. Consumers' lack of expertise regarding the health care alternatives facing them often results in health care decisions being made by providers.

   This set of related institutional arrangements has contributed to the current cost inflation in medical care. Furthermore, this inflation has affected both the public and the private sectors. In the public sector, fewer resources have been available to support the development of new social programs as less of the total budget becomes discretionary. In the private sector, health care cost inflation has reduced that part of the employee compensation package available for wages and other benefits and possibly increased the price of consumer goods as a result of the higher fringe benefit costs.

   This inflation has prompted two recent legislative proposals: the administration's Hospital Cost Containment Act of 1977 (HR 6575) and Senator Talmadge's Medicare and Medicaid Administrative and Reimbursement Reform Act (S 1470). The present analysis has two purposes: to evaluate these two proposals in terms of their impact on health care cost inflation and to make recommendations regarding a more satisfactory hospital cost containment program. The analysis presupposes that a cost containment program, effective in both the short and long run, should achieve the following objectives:

1. *To be consistent with a National Health Insurance (NHI) program.* The analysis provided here will neither assess the desirability of NHI nor evaluate alternative designs for such a program. It will, however, assess the effectiveness of the proposed cost containment programs in reducing the rate of increase in health care costs.
2. *To reduce the level of inefficiency in the health care system, for example, by reducing the number of underused beds and avoiding the duplication of services.*
3. *To alter the decisionmaking mechanisms and organization of the industry, to restructure incentives, and to alter the goals of providers in order to provide health care services that are appropriate at a reasonable cost.* While hospitals account for the largest single share of health care expenditures, effects on other providers indirectly affected by the legislation must also be considered.
4. *To permit learning from experience with a specific program so that it can be revised, improved, or possibly eliminated in light of that experience.* A cost containment program should be adaptive and adaptable so that performance can be used to guide future adjustments.

5. *To apply cost containment controls in a manner that offers a realistic likelihood for achieving results and to apply the controls to those components of the system most likely to yield cost savings.*
6. *To apply cost containment controls in as equitable a manner as possible.*
7. *To be consistent with, and to encourage, more fundamental reforms in insurance, organizational, and reimbursement arrangements, which may, at some future date, make direct cost controls unnecessary.*

HOSPITAL COST INFLATION

For an analysis of either the administration or the Talmadge proposal to be fully appreciated or for an alternative cost control program to be understood, the reader must first be aware of the nature of the cost inflation problem in the hospital industry. The rapid rate of hospital cost inflation in the past decade is a function of increases in the costs of factors that hospitals purchase to produce care and of increases in the number of services provided to each patient. For example, the American Hospital Association's Hospital Cost Index tracks the cost changes of a fixed set of thirty-seven services provided per typical patient day and their Hospital Intensity Index tracks changes in the quantities of the same thirty-seven services provided per typical patient day. From January 1976 to January 1977, the Hospital Cost Index increased 9.44 percent while the Hospital Intensity Index increased 6.13 percent.[1] (As a specific example of the increase in intensity phenomenon, Scitovsky and McCall found that from 1951 to 1964, in one hospital setting, the number of laboratory tests per case of perforated appendicitis increased from 5.3 to 14.5 and the number of postoperative intravenous solutions increased from 6.7 to 12.7 per case.)[2]

The figures suggest that if intensity stopped increasing, hospital cost increases would be about equal to the 9 percent target specified in the administration's cost containment proposal. While these intensity increases may contribute to improved quality of care, it is likely that comprehensive insurance coverage and the difficulty of making cost-quality tradeoffs at the system level encourage individuals and their physicians to use almost any service or treatment that might produce an improvement in the patient's health, no matter what the cost. In addition, technological innovation, which in the health field is often cost increasing rather than cost reducing, has been escalating at a very rapid rate. This escalation is not surprising given (1) the confidence of providers that they can generate the revenue needed to cover the cost of new services and technology, (2) the supply of new medical technology resulting from the profit objectives of suppliers, and (3) governmental and foundation support for biomedical research.

A great deal of attention has been focused recently on reducing inefficiency in the hospital industry. Inefficiency in individual hospitals, however, does not adequately explain the industrywide or systemwide inefficiency. The fundamental issue is not how well individual hospitals perform in efficiently providing services (although this is important), but rather the fact that the same level of services could be achieved if some of the components of the system were consolidated. Such consolidation would permit industry efficiency to be increased. The principal task of a cost containment proposal is therefore to provide the mechanisms for increasing industry efficiency by determining which components of the industry should remain and which should be consolidated.

EXPERIENCE WITH CONTROLS TO DATE

The administration and the Talmadge proposals are not the first to be suggested for controlling health care costs. An important program intended to reduce hospital cost inflation is prospective reimbursement—a program that has generally been supported by the hospital industry. There are many prospective rate-setting models, including complete review and negotiation of budgets, formula-based methods, and methods incorporating budget review by exception using cost and productivity screens to identify components of hospital costs that appear to be particularly out of line. The experience with prospective reimbursement to date is confounded by numerous exogenous factors. At best, these programs appear to have produced only small savings. Many of the difficulties in designing and administering a prospective reimbursement system concern the problem of measuring the product of a hospital, thereby making it difficult to establish a reimbursement rate. While budget review and negotiation may be an effective means of setting a rate when dealing with a limited number of hospitals, this kind of individualized approach to rate setting would be expensive, complex, and time consuming if implemented on a national level. Formulas for reimbursement, rather than an individual hospital approach, are central features of both the administration and the Talmadge proposals.

Certificate of need (CON) legislation is another major attempt to control hospital costs by limiting hospital capital expenditures. Without a control mechanism and with present forms of open-ended, third party reimbursement, there is likely to be excessive investment in the health care industry. Although CON programs have been established, their experience is limited and their impact to date mixed. While these programs may have had some effect on investment in bed capacity, hospitals appeared to have shifted their expansion objectives from beds to the acquisition of new equipment and medical technology. Moreover, since CON agencies have operated without an explicit limitation on the amount of capital expenditures and without a clear mechanism for determining need, it should not be surprising that only the form and not the magnitude of investment has been affected. While the administration's proposal places a much-needed limit on capital expenditure increases, the problem of evaluating alternatives for the limited expenditures on the basis of relative need is not addressed.

The most comprehensive experience with controls to date can be found in the Economic Stabilization Program. While the lessons from this program are often unclear, one of the clearest appears to be that if a cost containment program is to have long-term benefit to society, it must be permanent and must be believed to be permanent. The administration's proposal suffers in this regard from its "transitional" nature.

Another cost containment program is the Professional Standards Review Organization (PSRO) provision in PL 92–603. The aim of this law is to determine the appropriateness of hospitalization and to reduce length of hospital stay, thus encouraging physicians to use outpatient and extended care facilities. The mechanism for implementation is a detailed review procedure. While the point is still debatable, studies by the Institute of Medicine (IOM) and Gertman have not found that PSROs and utilization review appreciably reduce rising costs.[3,4] The IOM study concluded that there was no conclusive evidence that utilization review was cost effective. The study also questioned whether the medical care audit component of PSRO legislation was associated with significant improvements in the quality of care. Although utilization review was found to be associated with decreased length of stay, the fixed costs of maintaining a bed were found to be such that it appeared doubtful whether the savings were sufficient to cover the costs of the review process.

An interesting, controversial, and potentially cost-effective form of utilization review has recently been developed in the provision of surgical care—namely, the second opinion program. The central mechanism in such a program is an "independent" evaluation of a surgical case by a second surgeon. Experience with these programs to date has been limited, however, and further evaluation is necessary.

A final experience with cost control programs is that of Canada. Within the context of a national insurance program, provincial governments have been actively involved in negotiating budgets with individual hospitals. A definitive evaluation of the success of these programs is also still pending.

With these comments on the causes of hospital cost inflation, the objectives of a cost containment program, the nature of the hospital cost inflation problem, and the experiences with cost containment programs to date serving as background, attention can now be turned to the administration and the Talmadge proposals, with a view both to their strengths and weaknesses and to the recommendation of a proposal believed to address their deficiencies.

THE ADMINISTRATION'S PROPOSAL

The stated objective of the administration's proposal is "to curb the inflation in hospital costs, which is currently running far ahead of other prices, and to pave the way for more fundamental reform of the methods by which hospitals are paid and of the supply and distribution of health care services." The proposal states that two factors have led to the crisis in health care: "a third-party payment system that gives patients and their physicians little cause to consider hospital costs," and the fact that "third-party payers reimburse hospitals on the basis of whatever the hospitals state as their costs, or whatever price the hospital charges."[5] To deal with these market failures, the administration has proposed "a transitional program . . . to bring the increase in hospital costs more in line with price trends in the rest of the economy."[6] The program would apply to all "acute care and specialty hospitals" except chronic care institutions, new hospitals, HMO–funded hospitals, and federal hospitals. The administration's proposal would apply to inpatient services only. It contains two main components: (1) an "adjusted inpatient hospital revenue increase limit" and (2) a national limit on capital expenditures by hospitals.

One of the principal features of the proposal is a formula for the determination of the maximum allowable increase in a hospital's inpatient revenue. The formula limits a hospital's percentage revenue increase to a wholly exogenous number—the GNP deflator plus an allowance for increases in intensity applied uniformly to all hospitals. It does not, for example, reward a particular hospital for having a lower than average rate of cost increase in the previous year or penalize it for having a higher than average rate of cost increase. The formula is thus neutral with respect to hospitals that begin at different levels of expenditure. It does not attempt to rationalize variations in the current level of expenditure nor does it attempt to treat efficient or inefficient hospitals differently.

If applied in successive years, the only increases in intensity of services that would be permitted hospitals in the long run would be those that could be realized by increased productivity in the provision of the existing levels of services. Under this formula, over the long run, hospital expenditures would grow at a rate equal to the GNP deflator. As a consequence, the share of GNP devoted to hospital care would shrink as real GNP increased.

In designing any formula for limiting hospital revenue, a basic objective should be to permit hospitals to obtain revenue to cover cost increases that are beyond their control, such as increases in certain input prices, while requiring hospitals to control those costs that are subject to their discretion, such as the levels of intensity used to treat certain conditions and "negotiated" wage increases.

The administration's proposal contains two major adjustments for the inpatient revenue limit: the labor cost exemption and the admissions load adjustment. While the reason for the labor cost exemption (which is to apply only to nonsupervisory wage increases) may be political, there are two possible justifications for it. The first might be an objective that calls for a redistribution of income from relatively high income individuals to less highly paid individuals. It can be shown, however, that hospital nonsupervisory personnel currently earn at least as much as personnel of the same skill level could earn in alternative employment situations. Another justification is that, without this protection, lower paid nonsupervisory personnel may bear a disproportionate share of the cost containment controls.

The second major adjustment to the inpatient revenue increase limit is a method of responding to changes in the level of admissions. If the number of admissions for a hospital is within +2 percent to −6 percent of the base year, the permitted increase in total inpatient revenue is equal to the allowable limit (e.g., 9 percent) applied to the base year revenue. (For smaller hospitals, admissions may fall by 10 percent without reducing revenue.) This implies that, for admission changes within these limits, revenue per admission will increase by less than 9 percent if admissions rise and will increase by more than 9 percent if admissions fall. If admissions increase by more than 2 percent, hospitals will receive for each extra admission 50 percent of base period revenue per admission. If admissions decrease by more than 6 percent, revenue is reduced by 50 percent of base period revenue per admission for each admission below 6 percent. These adjustments are limited to a ±15 percent change in admissions interval.

While the administration's proposal is temporary and is directed at controlling short-run costs, volume changes ultimately have long-run effects. Long-run decreases in volume should lead to decreases in available beds, reductions in services that can be more economically provided at other hospitals, and reductions in personnel at both the supervisory and nonsupervisory levels. Long-run incremental costs are closer to average costs than are short-term incremental costs, and certainly are higher than the 50 percent figure specified for changes outside the −6 to +2 percent corridor. As a result, application of the formula in successive years would not be consistent with the long-run cost structure of hospitals. Hospitals with increasing admissions may not be able to generate sufficient revenue to cover the cost of providing the greater level of care within the 50 percent limit, while hospitals with decreasing admissions should be able to reduce costs more than the 50 percent reduction imposed on them. The short- and long-run effects of the formula are thus quite different. These observations point to the desirability of instituting a long-term policy rather than a series of short-run policies which, while they may function effectively in the short run, would in the long run create an excessive burden on hospitals in the growing areas and a windfall for hospitals that permanently reduce output.

The Outpatient Care Exemption
A feature of the administration's proposal that deserves careful attention is the exemption of outpatient revenues from controls. To predict the effects of this exemption, it is important to realize that outpatient departments of hospitals serve two roles. In part, they are complementary to the hospital's inpatient care, since some procedures that relate to an inpatient hospital episode can be performed in outpatient departments either before or after the hospitalization. On the other hand, however, outpatient departments are substitutes both for inpatient care and for physician office practices. The extremely rapid growth of hospital outpatient visits is primarily the result of the substitution of hospital services for physician office services. For families in low income neighborhoods, particularly, the hospital outpatient department is often the main source of primary care.

It is likely that the exemption of outpatient care would increase the demand for outpatient care and consequently the price of that care. Substitution of outpatient for inpatient care seems generally desirable and would be encouraged by the exemption. If hospitals turn to their outpatient departments to increase revenue and expand services, however, this exemption may not be expedient. There may also be a temptation to use the flexibility of accounting procedures to shift revenues from inpatient to outpatient accounts. Instead of exempting outpatient services from controls, it would be better to devise a formula that would allow hospitals to choose the mix of inpatient and outpatient services that is appropriate.

Limitation on Capital Expenditures

To avoid duplication of services and to limit the expenditure for new technology, the administration's proposal contains a program designed to limit hospital capital expenditures by imposing a national limit on such expenditures. While a national limit on capital expenditures may well be necessary, there are two primary problems associated with the limit. First, the $2.5 billion upper limit is arbitrary. The present state of knowledge probably does not permit an explicit determination of a "best" limit, but the proposal would be improved if it included a mechanism that allowed the level to be an explicit object of collective choice. That choice could reflect a comparison, at the collective level, of social benefits and costs. This comparison could be made by Health Systems Agencies (HSAs) and local certificate of need agencies. They are not currently staffed to play this demanding role, however. Accordingly, provision should be made in the proposal for increases in the capacity of these agencies. The second problem in administering the capital expenditures program lies in the exclusionary provisions based on the current bed supply in a community and on the current occupancy rate. These restrictions come very close to preventing any new investment in beds. Based upon information in the 1975 *Hospital Guide Issue*, these restrictions would prevent investment in new beds in all but two of the one hundred largest cities.[7] Fifty-eight of these one hundred cities have an occupancy rate below 80 percent. All but two of those with occupancy rates over 80 percent, however, have greater than four beds per 1,000 population. Similarly, 244 of 297 standard metropolitan statistical areas would be unable to invest in beds. In addition, in forty-eight of the fifty states plus the District of Columbia, the occupancy for nonmetropolitan areas is below 80 percent (the exceptions are New York and New Jersey). The capital expenditures limit should, therefore, be flexible enough to permit latitude for special situations.

THE TALMADGE PROPOSAL

The major innovative feature of the Talmadge proposal is a mechanism for incentive reimbursement for "routine operating hospital costs" for Medicare and Medicaid patients. This incentive reimbursement mechanism may be appropriate if the cause of the high level of hospital costs is cost or technical inefficiency in hospitals, presumably in the form of excess beds, excessive staffing, and other forms of duplication. The mechanism is intended to reward those hospitals that have costs lower than the average for their classification while not penalizing those hospitals whose costs are higher than the average for their class. These hospital classifications are to be developed by the Secretary of Health, Education and Welfare. Specifically, a hospital that experiences per diem routine operating costs that are below the per diem payment rate established for its hospital class would be reimbursed for its actual costs plus an incentive payment equal to 50 percent of the difference between the payment rate and the actual cost, with a limit on the incentive payment equal to 5 percent of the payment rate. Thus, when costs are below the established payment rate, the hospital and the government share the benefits equally. When costs are in excess of the payment rate, reimbursement would be made for costs up to 120 percent of the payment rate.

This incentive mechanism appears to be based on the assumption that a hospital will try to increase net revenues by lowering its costs below its group average through reductions in inefficiency. Such behavior would be more difficult for those hospitals that are already efficient but have high costs for other reasons, such as case mix, than it would be for those hospitals that are inefficient. The mechanism could also reward some inefficient hospitals, namely, those hospitals that are inefficient but have costs that are below the average for their group because of reasons, such as case mix or low service intensity, that are not considered in the classification mechanisms. Even if such hospitals experienced a very high rate of increase in costs or became somewhat more inefficient, they could still qualify for the incentive payment.

As suggested above, however, there is little evidence that variation across hospitals in routine costs can be attributed to inefficiency. Thus, it seems unlikely that a strategy designed essentially to increase individual institutional efficiency will solve the larger issue of rapidly escalating health care costs.

Another important feature of the Talmadge proposal is an exemption for ancillary services. If major causes of the rapid hospital inflation are excessive rates both of expansion in hospital services and of acquisition of medical technology, however, this exemption removes any deterrent to the rate of increase in these costs. Indeed, the exemption may contribute to inflation of ancillary costs as hospitals shift their expansion and growth objectives toward such services. While the expansion of these services might have health care enhancement effects, this exemption allows hospitals and third party payers to avoid facing the real issue of the cost-quality tradeoff associated with expanded services.

The bill also exempts from coverage energy expenses and malpractice insurance costs. These exemptions are appropriate because these costs are basically beyond the control of the hospital and would confound the classification scheme. The costs associated with educational and training programs are also exempt, since such programs presumably are desired by society primarily for their educational benefits, not for their immediate effects on the cost of hospital care.

Also exempted from coverage under the per diem payment rate is the cost of "nonadministrative physicians." One recent trend in hospitals is the expansion of their salaried medical staff. This expansion increases hospital-billed costs, but it may not involve a substantial increase in health care costs because fee for service billings may be correspondingly reduced. A danger in this exemption, however, is that hospitals may decide to allocate additional resources to their salaried medical staff in excess of the level needed to provide the appropriate level of care. The motivation for such action would be the same as that for the expansion of services, since an expanded medical staff adds prestige to a hospital.

TECHNICAL ISSUES IN
COST CONTAINMENT

With the overview of the administration and the Talmadge proposals as background, several technical issues that any cost containment program must address can be discussed. A central problem in any attempt to control costs in the hospital industry is that of how to compare hospitals. It is possible to group or classify them according to a number of variables including size, types of cases treated, and so forth. The effectiveness of any cost containment program will depend on how well such a grouping is accomplished. The criteria on which a classification system can be evaluated include (1) its consideration of the factors that determine the types of hospital service, (2) its degree of differentiation of hospitals that produce different services, (3) the extent to which it captures the structural relationship between hospital characteristics and type of service output, (4) its equity in the eyes of providers, (5) its ease of administration, and (6) its resistance to easy manipulation by providers for their own purposes. A classification system satisfying all of these criteria is clearly difficult to devise.

Another important consideration in designing a cost containment program is the problem of anticipation. If hospitals anticipated that controls were to be introduced, they might take actions to weaken the ultimate impact of the controls. To avoid such an anticipation effect, the administration's proposal develops its revenue base from past data: "The base would be the dollar total of the hospital's revenue from each class of payer for calendar 1976. . . ." The rationale for this approach is stated as follows: "This method would assure that any hospital which raised charges after public announcement of the Administration's hospital cost containment effort would not benefit from that action."[8]

The Talmadge proposal does not directly deal with this anticipation effect. In that proposal, the groupings of hospitals are likely to be sufficiently large so that no individual hospital could significantly affect the average, but if all hospitals anticipated the controls in some manner, the average could be altered substantially. The Talmadge proposal appears to invite this type of anticipatory effect by stating: "FY1978 cost data would be used in developing a listing of payment rates . . . on an advisory and informational basis only. FY1979 data, based on the accounting and uniform reporting system, would be used in determining the payment rates to be fully effective in FY1981."[9] The use of 1979 data allows hospitals ample time to expand services and costs in anticipation of the incentive reimbursement mechanism. The administration's approach to lessening the impact of anticipatory responses by basing allowable revenue limits on past (1976) data may be a better approach than that of the Talmadge proposal. The principal policy implication of the anticipation problem is that a regulatory proposal for cost containment should be contemplated only as a long-term policy, so that the effect of any preemptive strategic behavior would be overshadowed by later years of effective regulation. A second implication is that a transitional program would influence the behavior of the industry toward a future program and would tend to promote strategic behavior to frustrate similar legislation in the future.

A third important consideration for cost containment proposals is the necessity of establishing a uniform cost accounting system. Such a uniform system is particularly necessary in conjunction with both the administration and the Talmadge bill because they both exempt certain types of services from controls. In the administration's bill, for example, outpatient services are exempt. Accordingly, one possible way in which hospitals could reduce their "costs subject to control" would be to allocate a greater amount of the common costs to outpatient services. Such reallocations would reduce the effectiveness of the controls.

CONSTRAINTS, REFORMS, AND
RATIONAL POLITICAL CHOICE

In view of the rather discouraging history of health care price controls and in view of the even more discouraging history of similar controls in other part of the economy, it may seem illogical to suggest greater government control as a solution to hospital cost inflation. An optimist may believe that there is light at the end of the regulatory tunnel and that some reforms in the regulatory process could improve matters. Other than optimism itself, however, there seems no reason to conclude that regulation in the future will work much better than regulation in the past. Why, then, should regulation be considered?

Market control in the hospital sector is presently imperfect because existing forms of insurance permit an individual or his physician to initiate actions that provide direct benefits to him without his having to bear more than a small fraction of the cost of these actions. If decisions were made governmentally, one may argue that, at least at the collective level, the cost of providing additional benefits would have to be faced. Although a consumer may be able to avoid the costs of his actions individually, he cannot avoid those costs collectively. Since existing insurance makes it impossible for costs and benefits to be compared individually, decisions may be able to be made more rationally (though surely not perfectly) if costs and benefits were compared collectively. Governmental or regulatory decisions will not be "perfect" because collective choice inherently fails to take full account of individual preferences and because incentive structures to induce regulators to perform well do not exist. One may hope, however, that some collective control, even if imperfect, would be better than the present open-ended system. Use of the market and use of regulation are two alternative forms of cost control. It is, however, a grave mistake to view them as necessarily mutually exclusive.

In addition to combining both in our approach to hospital cost containment, it would also appear appropriate to address more fundamental reforms in insurance, organization, or reimbursement that hold the promise of leading to better comparison of costs and benefits. The regulatory controls that will be discussed, even in their final (as opposed to transitional) forms, should not be viewed as the only, or even necessarily as the most important, way of controlling hospital costs. They are rather a safety net, intended to catch the system while more fundamental reforms take time to work or temporarily do not work. Eventually, the regulatory constraints might not be binding, at least not for many hospitals or many parts of the country. Fundamental reforms, such as indemnity insurance, HMOs and other procompetitive arrangements, greater use of consumer cost sharing, and cost control efforts such as preadmission screening, surgical second opinion programs, and utilization review are certainly not precluded by the existence of upper limits on costs. It should be made clear that these limits are not floors but ceilings, which would permit well-managed hospitals to continue to perform in a way that provided a standard for their less well-managed counterparts.

Chapter 2

Outline of a Recommended
Cost Containment Program

INTRODUCTION

A hospital cost containment program and a set of recommendations for long-term reform are outlined below. The proposed program takes into account the magnitude and complexity of the problem of hospital cost inflation. It also deals with the problems identified in the administration and the Talmadge proposals and builds on their strengths. Although some of the details of this suggested program, such as the administrative mechanism and the implementation procedures, still remain to be developed, the following sections describe its broad features.

Since the primary dimensions of the hospital cost inflation problem are the rapid increase in service intensity, inefficiency at the industry level, and the inability and/or unwillingness of providers to make explicit cost-quality tradeoffs, the recommended program is designed to encourage and induce both hospital decisionmakers and local and state planners to focus on these problems. The recommended program incorporates national controls on both revenue and capital expenditures as constraints under which decisionmakers are to exercise their judgment and authority. These two forms of controls are to be parallel in design and in administration so that more effective planning can take place. The parallel between the revenue limitation and the capital expenditure control features of the proposed program would permit coordination at the local level, so that authorized capital expenditures for expanded services could be matched by allowed increases in revenue to cover the operating costs incurred in utilizing those services.

17

While these controls are to be established on a national basis, the allocation of allowable increases and expenditures among hospitals would be made at the local level. An important feature of the program is that HSAs and state planning agencies would be required to submit an annual report to the Secretary of Health, Education and Welfare that explicitly documented expected improvements in consumer health and well-being that could be achieved in their areas if their revenue and capital expenditure allocations were to be increased. This would then give planners at the federal level some basis for estimating an "opportunity value" that could be used to judge the desirability of increased revenue or capital expenditure allocations to particular areas. In addition to providing information for use at the national level, the cost containment program proposed here would cause state and local agencies to compete with one another. They would have the incentive to seek out and document those local hospital programs and service expansions that could provide the greatest improvements in the quality, comprehensiveness, and distribution of health care in their communities. This aspect of the cost containment program thus provides part of a mechanism for dealing, in an admittedly imprecise manner, with both the determination of an appropriate national rate of increase in hospital costs and the allocation of that increase among the states and among the HSAs. The specifics of this hospital cost containment program are outlined in the following sections.

THE PROPOSED HOSPITAL COST CONTAINMENT PROGRAM

Limitations on Revenue

Item 1. National Revenue Limitation. *A national revenue limit shall be applied to both inpatient and outpatient programs of a hospital. The limit shall be based on a formula containing two basic components: (a) an allowed revenue increase equal to the GNP deflator and (b) an allowed increase in revenue determined by the Secretary, to permit increases in intensity and expansion of hospital services. This latter increase would be limited to 3 percent in the first two years of the program and in future years would be adapted to the demonstrated needs for expanded hospital care programs and services. The total allowed increase in revenue would be applied to each third party cost payer and to individual payers.*

Rationale

1. A revenue limit places the obligation and decisionmaking authority for hospital cost containment with hospital administrators, physicians, and trustees by requiring them to operate within a revenue limit.

2. Since the prices that hospitals pay for labor and the other inputs that they employ are to some degree exogenous and beyond their control, hospitals should be permitted to pass these higher input prices on to consumers. The GNP deflator may be preferred to a hospital-specific input price index because wage rate increases may have an endogenous component and because suppliers to the hospital industry may exercise some degree of oligopolistic pricing power. The use of the GNP deflator may encourage hospitals to exercise countervailing power against suppliers of inputs. Exceptions to this provision are contained in Item 6.

3. Since some expansion of hospital programs and some increase in service intensity would appear to be warranted, an allowance is provided for revenue increases to cover the resulting additional costs. Since the optimal level of such cost increases is not known, a reasonable starting point would be to set them to maintain the present proportion of GNP devoted to hospital care. The 3 percent figure for the first two years is chosen as an approximation of the average annual increase in real GNP, so that hospital costs would remain approximately at the present percentage of GNP. The hospital system would be able to expand programs and services beyond the 3 percent limit to the extent that productivity could be improved, and the gains could be allocated to expansion and increases in intensity. Consequently, if average hospital productivity increased by 2 percent annually, service intensity could be increased by 5 percent. This feature provides an incentive for increases in productivity.

4. Inpatient and outpatient revenue would be covered by the revenue limit, so that hospitals would be required to make judgments on the appropriate mix of inpatient and outpatient services. This uniform coverage would also avoid accounting manipulations designed to circumvent controls. Item 4 describes revenue adjustments for the level of both inpatient and outpatient services.

5. Educational and training programs would be covered, so that hospitals would be required to determine whether the long-range benefits of these programs warrant the associated cost. If it were thought that hospitals might disproportionately reduce desirable outpatient programs or desirable educational activities in order to stay under the revenue limit, it would be possible to give special treatment to these activities. Outpatient department revenues might be

permitted to increase more rapidly than inpatient revenues, and increased educational and training costs could be reason for an exemption from the revenue ceiling.

Item 2. Allocation of the National Revenue Limit to HSAs. *The national revenue limitation shall be allocated to HSAs based on adjustments for the nature and role of the hospitals in the HSA. As a basis for the allocation, the Secretary shall devise an appropriate classification system for hospitals, taking into account parameters such as (a) the licensed number of beds of the hospital; (b) the approved programs of the hospital, including teaching programs, research programs, and community service programs; (c) the size of the SMSA in which the hospital is located; (d) the census region in which the hospital is located; and (e) any other parameters that the Secretary judges to be appropriate. The Secretary would be charged with determining which dimensions should be used to classify hospitals.*

The average percentage increase in revenue over the 1975–1977 fiscal year period for each class will be determined by the Secretary. The average increase over all hospitals in the country is not to exceed the national limit established in Item 1. In no event would a hospital class receive an allowable limit below that of the GNP deflator. The total revenue increase allocated to an HSA shall then be determined by aggregating the allowed revenue increase for each hospital in the HSA by class.

Rationale

1. Hospitals perform differing functions in the health care system, and these role differences should be recognized as having differing cost implications. An initial hospital classification system is thus recommended based both on hospital-specific characteristics—that is, bed size and programs—as well as on exogenous factors such as geographic location and the urban or rural environment of the hospital. Classification by hospital-specific characteristics allows for differences in the scope of services provided by hospitals, while classification by SMSA size and census region allows for increases in costs due to (a) differential rates of increase of wage rates and (b) differential rates of growth of population and, hence, of hospital admissions. The classification of hospitals according to approved programs is meant to be a readily implementable surrogate for case mix. Since the number of approved programs or facilities is not a perfect proxy for case mix, the Secretary shall be charged with developing a classification scheme based on actual case mix differences.

2. The relative percentage increase in cost for each hospital class is also to be determined by the Secretary. It may be that increases in service intensity are more desirable for some types of hospitals than for others or that there are regional differences in the rate of increase in input prices.

Item 3. Allocation of the HSA Allowed Revenue Increase Among Hospitals. *The authority for the allocation of the allowed revenue increase among hospitals shall reside at the state level, and the allocation shall be approved by a "State Health Reimbursement Board" according to criteria it deems appropriate. The composition of and criteria for membership on this board remain to be determined. Likewise, criteria for allocation need to be determined but may include those used in Item 2, as well as any potential effects on community health, the extent to which the hospital provides primary care to an underserved population, service expansion requirements, occupancy rates, and so forth. No hospital shall be granted a revenue increase limit less than that indicated by the GNP deflator.*

While final authority rests at the state level, the local HSAs shall be responsible for determining priorities among revenue increase requests from different hospitals and for preparing recommendations for allocating the allowed increase among the hospitals within its jurisdiction. At the end of each fiscal year, each HSA and each state is required to submit an annual report to the Secretary stating the criteria used for the allocation among hospitals and detailing the actions that would have been taken in its area had its allowed revenue increase been greater by 1 percent, by 2 percent, by 3 percent, and by 4 percent (i.e., 9 percent + 4 percent). The HSA will develop this latter part of the report in conjunction with the hospitals and other providers in its area.

Rationale

1. Not only do hospitals perform differing roles in the health care delivery system, but different communities and regions also have differing health care needs. Consequently, a national formula for all hospitals is not sensitive enough to differing roles and needs to provide for an appropriate allocation of health care expenditures among hospitals. This allocation can better be made at the local HSA level than at the national level. Furthermore, states and HSAs are asked to develop the criteria that they feel are appropriate for their particular situations.

2. The required annual report will permit the Secretary to review the criteria used, but more importantly, will indicate the value of

additional incremental allocations to an HSA. This feature encourages competition among HSAs to develop proposals for the best additions to their health care delivery system and allows the Secretary to determine the merit of adjusting the social budget for the allowed increase for expansion and intensity specified in Item 1.

Item 4. Adjustment for Changes in Admissions. *The allowed revenue increase for a hospital as determined under the provisions of Item 3 shall be adjusted based on the relationship between the current level of adjusted admissions and the 1976 base year adjusted admissions. The adjusted admissions for a hospital shall be determined by adding to admissions the number of outpatient visits multiplied by a weighting factor. Initially, this factor will be the hospital's ratio of outpatient revenue per visit to inpatient revenue per admission. Ultimately, with appropriate cost accounting methods, it will be based on relative costs. The payment rate utilized in the adjustments is the average revenue per adjusted admission for the previous year increased by the allowable revenue increase for that hospital as determined in Item 3. Revenues will be increased by 30 percent of the payment rate for each additional adjusted admission if adjusted admissions in the current year are above those in the base year 1976 but are less than 1.02 of the base year's adjusted admissions. Revenues will be decreased by 30 percent of the payment rate for each adjusted admission for adjusted admissions decreases that are less than 6 percent of the base year's adjusted admissions. If adjusted admissions increase by at least 2 percent, a revenue increase will be granted, for each adjusted admission above the 2 percent level, equal to 60 percent of the payment rate. For adjusted admission decreases beyond −6 percent, a revenue deduction will be made equal to 40 percent of the payment rate. Hospitals with 1976 admissions below 4,000 shall use a lower limit of −10 percent rather than −6 percent.*

Rationale

1. Since hospital admissions are to a substantial extent beyond the control of an individual hospital, revenue increases should be permitted for any significant changes in the level of admissions. The −6 percent to +2 percent corridor is intended to pertain to adjustments due to random fluctuations in admissions, and the 30 percent cost allowance is intended to reflect short-run costs such as supplies that would vary with the level of admissions. The corridor is wider on the downside, since it is more difficult to make short-term adjustments in response to admissions decreases than it is to adjust to increases in admissions. The specific limits on the corridor are arbitrary, and the

Secretary shall examine the limits to determine more appropriate limits.

2. An admissions basis is used instead of a patient day basis because admissions are less controllable by hospitals than are patient days.

3. Adjusted admissions is used as a base in order not to create any unwarranted incentives or disincentives for the use of outpatient services. The adjustment formula determines an "outpatient visit equivalent" admission based on a revenue ratio, so a hospital that shifts from inpatient care to outpatient care will not be penalized so long as the revenue difference between inpatient and outpatient care is proportional to the cost difference. The use of adjusted admissions avoids the need to exempt outpatient services in order to encourage increased use of outpatient care.

4. The 60 percent figure is set at a level between the short-run variable cost percentage of average cost, estimated to be approximately 30 percent, and the long-run incremental cost percentage, estimated to be about 90 percent based on econometric estimates that indicate slightly increasing returns for hospitals. Although the cost containment program is to be permanent, the long-run incremental cost figure is not used because that value may include the effects of expansions in services and service intensity for which a separate allowance has been made in Item 1. The 40 percent figure is used because it is more difficult to adjust to decreases in admissions than to increases. Research to determine a more precise measure of long-run cost that does not include the effect of increased service intensity is needed.

5. The 1976 adjusted admissions base is used in order to permit revenue adjustments for admissions changes that occur over time but are within the corridor in any year. For example, if admissions at a hospital increase 1 percent a year, the hospital would be permitted the 60 percent revenue increase on the initial 1 percent growth in the third year and in successive years.

6. A wider corridor is used for smaller hospitals, since they are more likely to experience greater percentage fluctuations in admissions.

Item 5. Differences Between Revenue and Cost. *If a hospital incurs cost increases for Medicare and Medicaid patients that are less than the revenue limit established in Items 3 and 4, the hospital shall receive an incentive payment equal to 50 percent of the excess of revenue limit over actual costs for these patients. The Secretary shall investigate the possibility of extending an incentive reimbursement* *mechanism to other third party payers. The Secretary shall also investigate the possibility of a common method of reimbursement for all patients.*

Rationale

In order to provide an additional incentive for cost containment at the level of the individual hospital, hospitals will be permitted to retain half of any excess they generate on Medicare and Medicaid transactions.

Item 6. Exceptions to the Revenue Limitations. *(a) The Secretary shall monitor the impact of the cost containment program on individual cost items in order to determine if any input, such as labor, is being unduly discriminated against. The Secretary shall be permitted to grant relief for those inputs that are being unduly penalized.*

Rationale

During Phase II of the Economic Stabilization Program, wage rates were effectively controlled, while other input prices were not. This regulation placed an unfair burden on hospital employees. If, in response to the cost containment program, hospitals place the burden of cost reductions primarily on employees, the Secretary can provide relief by adjusting the revenue limit for additional increases in labor costs.

(b) The Secretary shall be empowered to make adjustments in the revenue limit for extraordinary exogenous increases in the price of any hospital input.

Rationale

This provision will avoid penalizing hospitals for extraordinary cost increases, such as for malpractice insurance, that are beyond their control. This provision will apply only to extraordinary occurrences, since the overall increase in input prices is considered in the GNP deflator in Item 1.

(c) Hospitals in a given state shall be exempt from the above provisions if the state has a comprehensive cost containment program that is at least as effective as the national program. A program shall be considered to be at least as effective as the national program if it limits total revenue increases for all hospitals in the state to a targeted amount less than or equal to the national revenue limits.

Rationale

Since states are major payers of hospital costs through Medicaid and other systems, a state may wish to control costs more stringently than the national program, and it should be permitted to do so.

(d) Insolvency: The Secretary shall be empowered to grant an exception to the revenue limit if it is deemed warranted for a hospital whose solvency is threatened by the revenue limitation.

Rationale

A hospital might find itself in a circumstance in which the application of the revenue limit might result in its insolvency. Petition for relief could be made by the responsible HSA and state agency. The petition would not be approved if closing of the hospital were determined to be appropriate.

Item 7. Requirements. *(a) A uniform accounting and reporting system shall be established for all hospitals. In developing such a system, the Secretary shall consult interested and knowledgeable parties, so that the reporting system would provide the required information with the least disruption in hospital administrative procedures. The accounting system should identify those costs associated with patient care, research, and teaching. It should also identify meaningful measures of intermediate outputs and patient characteristics.*

Rationale

Such a uniform system is necessary to monitor performance, to permit HSAs and state agencies to make allocations among hospitals, and to facilitate a closer approximation of the direct costs of patient care, research, and teaching.

(b) Hospitals shall be required to maintain their present share of charity cases.

Rationale

Since the purpose of the cost containment program is to induce hospitals to provide care at lower resource cost, hospitals should not be permitted to stay within the revenue limit by reducing care to charity patients and using the resources thus saved to provide more costly care to other patients.

(c) The Secretary shall monitor changes in physician compensation and physician staffing within the hospital and adjust the revenue limit if hospitals attempt to shift costs currently included in the hospital budget to fee for service billing. If physicians are converted from a fee for service billing basis to a salaried position, the Secretary may increase the revenue limit accordingly.

Rationale

Hospitals have an opportunity to reduce their costs by shifting radiologists, pathologists, anesthesiologists, and other physicians from a salaried basis to a fee for service billing basis. If this occurs, the Secretary is required to reduce the hospital's revenue limit commensurately. Opposite shifts that may reduce health care system costs would warrant revenue increases.

Capital Expenditure Controls

Item 8. The National Limit. *Each year the Secretary shall determine, based on need, an amount of capital expenditures to be authorized for the hospital sector, not to exceed $2.5 billion annually for the first two years of the program. The authorized amount shall be divided into two parts: (a) $1.5 billion to be allocated to states solely on the basis of population, and (b) $1.0 billion to be allocated to states on the basis of their proposals for capital expenditures. During the first year of the program, the total amount shall be distributed solely on the basis of population. The amounts will be proportionately reduced if the Secretary sets an expenditure limit below $2.5 billion. In making the allocations from the second part, the Secretary may take into account construction costs, demographic changes, the existing number of beds per capita, occupancy rates, the distribution of health services among socioeconomic groups, expenditures required for compliance with health and safety requirements, and so forth. No expenditure shall be authorized from the second pool for bed expansion if there are at least four beds per 1,000 population in an HSA or where the occupancy rate in an HSA is less than 80 percent. The authorization for capital expenditures is to cover all spending for construction and equipment purchases in excess of $100,000.*

Rationale

1. A capital expenditure limit is needed to require planners and providers to address the health care gains that can be achieved through capital additions. While the $2.5 billion limit is arbitrary and

may warrant alteration in the future, this value is about half the current rate of expenditure and would necessitate allocations among competing alternatives. Hospitals, HSAs, and state agencies would be required to choose between bed expansion and the acquisition of technology.

2. The authorized amount would be divided into two pools, the larger of which would be allocated solely on the basis of population, so that all states might expand their investment in hospital facilities and equipment as they deemed appropriate. The second pool would be allocated among the states by the Secretary on the basis of the improvements in health care anticipated to result from the capital authorization.

3. The administration's bed and occupancy ratio criteria are arbitrary. If they were believed to be appropriate national goals, however, they could be applied to the discretionary pool.

4. All sources of capital are to be covered by this system, so that hospitals with access to a variety of sources of funds would not be able to circumvent the controls.

Item 9. State Allocation of the Capital Expenditure Authorization. *In conjunction with hospitals under their jurisdiction, HSAs shall be responsible for aggregating and indicating priorities for capital expenditure proposals and making recommendations regarding their funding. An HSA shall coordinate the capital expenditure proposals with its revenue increase recommendations. These recommendations are to be transmitted for final decision to the state agency charged with administering the certificate of need program. The state shall then make detailed proposals to the Secretary for projects to be funded from the second discretionary pool.*

Rationale

1. As with the allocation of revenue increases, the HSA is best able to develop priorities for the capital needs of hospitals in its area. This process will guide the state agency in its allocation and will assist the Secretary in determining the appropriate budget for capital expenditure.

2. By having an HSA recommend which capital expenditures should be made, it will be able to coordinate the capital expenditure program with the revenue increase allocation. It may be desirable to increase a hospital's revenue limit so that it will be able to obtain the revenue to cover the costs incurred in operating the new facilities or providing the new services without having to reduce some other activity.

Item 10. Decertification. *A local HSA shall be responsible for preparing recommendations for the decertification of technology, services, and facilities for hospitals in its area in order to provide a more rational allocation of resources among hospitals. Such recommendations shall be considered by the state certificate of need agency, and if approved, the technology, service, or facility shall be discontinued. The HSA shall coordinate decertification decisions with its revenue increase recommendations. Any costs associated with service termination, initiated either by an HSA or a hospital, will result in an equivalent adjustment in the hospital's revenue limit.*

Rationale

1. The capital expenditure controls are designed both to place a limit on and to rationally distribute the expansion of technology, services, and facilities. In a recent report, entitled *Hospital Regulation: Report of the Special Committee on the Regulatory Process*, the American Hospital Association has recognized the passive nature of previous planning mechanisms and the need for new methods to deal with technology, services, and facilities that are in excess supply.[1]

2. The local HSA is best able to evaluate community needs. It would appear to be best able to make knowledgeable decisions about decertification.

3. In order that costs associated with the termination of services did not impose a burden on a hospital, an additional revenue increase would be permitted. This revenue increase would also encourage hospitals to terminate services subject to certificate of need agency approval as required by PL 93−641.

IMPLEMENTATION

Decisions on the allocation of funds at the federal, state, and HSA level will obviously be difficult and will require a level of information, resources, and expertise not presently available at any of these levels. Indeed, except for those states with rate review boards, appropriate state agencies probably do not now exist. In addition, given the past history of regulation in general, and of regulation in health in particular, the eventual success of these proposed regulatory efforts is by no means assured.

These observations suggest that it would be necessary to have a transitional period before the above recommendations could be fully implemented. In this transitional period, somewhat arbitrary allocations would have to substitute for rational planning, and these allocations would have to be carefully monitored. Given that service intensity may in many instances be in excess of that warranted by a comparison of benefits and costs, it is anticipated that restrictions in the increase in service intensity would have little serious adverse short-run consequences for the health or well-being of consumers.

Rather than moving precipitously from arbitrary rules of thumb to the regulation scheme described above, it may be preferable to adjust gradually the amount of increase in revenue permitted each hospital. One way of accomplishing this task would be to gradually reduce the proportion of each hospital's allowable percentage increase in inpatient revenue that was determined by rules of thumb and to gradually increase the portion determined by rationalized planning.

HSAs play a critical role in our recommended cost containment program. As noted previously, they are currently underequipped to perform the role required of them. In order for them to perform this role, their resources—staff, budgets, and data inputs—would have to be significantly increased. Of even greater importance, HSAs would have to devise, or have devised for them, the principles and methods for measuring the benefits of various "quality improvements" proposed by hospitals in their areas and for evaluating them against their costs. The rate at which each HSA could evolve from rules of thumb to rational planning would depend on their relative success in generating resources and in developing and applying the appropriate analytic framework.

LONG-TERM REFORM

The hospital cost containment program described above provides mechanisms to control the rate of increase in hospital costs, but it does not remedy the fundamental causes of the problem, addressed in the next section of this book. There are, however, a number of steps that should be taken to address the deficiencies present in the health care marketplace. Successful resolution of these deficiencies could eventually facilitate the dismantling of the cost containment program with the confidence that natural incentives could provide for an appropriate level of health care expenditures in line with the value placed on that care by consumers.

Restructuring of the Insurance System

A major cause of hospital cost inflation is the present nature of insurance coverage. On the whole, hospitalization insurance does not give consumers an incentive to choose among health care providers on the basis of cost and quality. This deficiency is compounded by the limited ability of consumers to judge quality differences. Programs to increase consumers' capacity to assess quality should be initiated, and consumers should be encouraged to become aware of cost differences among providers. To foster this latter goal, two mechanisms that warrant further study, particularly in light of a national health insurance plan, are indemnity plans and provider fee schedules.

Indemnity plans take a variety of forms. Their general characteristic is that the consumer chooses an insurance with a maximum payment level per unit. If he elects a provider whose cost and charge is higher than this maximum, he will have to bear the cost of that choice. For example, Newhouse and Taylor have proposed an arrangement, called variable cost insurance, in which a person who chooses insurance also selects the type of hospital in which he would prefer to be treated.[2] All hospitals in the person's area are classified by an "expense rating," so that if he selects a more expensive hospital, he will have to pay a higher premium. If the hospital actually used is no more expensive than his expense class, his expenses would be covered in full. If, however, a more expensive hospital is used, he would have to pay some part of the incremental costs. Premiums would, of course, be lower, the lower the level of costliness selected. A similar idea (generalized to include physician costs and total expense as well) has been presented by Ellwood and McClure under the notion of "Health Care Alliances."[3] Here, the insurance company specifies a particular set of physicians who will provide care and ties the premium to the expenses generated by the physicians in the alliance. The consumer would be able to choose from competing alliances offered by several insurance firms. In either case, the consumer is able to retain extensive insurance coverage, but there is a stronger incentive to providers to become or remain efficient, while at the same time permitting consumers who prefer high cost providers to use these services if they are willing to pay the cost of doing so.

Fee schedules for providers can be a form of indemnity if the provider is permitted to bill for more than the fee schedule level. If the provider must accept the fee schedule as payment in full, but may refuse to provide service, then the consumer has an incentive to search for providers whose costs are not in excess of the fee schedule maximum. Finally, and most importantly, if additional billing is not permitted and if providers accept the fee schedule payments, that schedule can be structured to serve as an incentive for the delivery of appropriate care. Adjustments in price would also help to control supply.

Supply Incentives

A second major cause of hospital cost inflation is the acquisition and utilization by hospitals of new medical technology. The rate of technological innovation is spurred by profit objectives of private companies and by federal support for biomedical research. Most of this innovation is directed at service improvement or product enhancement, and there is little incentive for providers of health care to choose among alternative new technologies so long as the costs can be completely recovered. Given this natural tendency, additional research funds should be marked for stimulating cost-reducing innovation that would permit hospitals, for example, to provide the same quality of care but at a reduced cost. In a similar way, decisions on governmental support of biomedical research and innovation should take the cost as well as the benefits of implementing successful research into account.

Quality of Care

To address the problem of measuring the gains in the quality of care associated with increased health care expenditures, a major effort should be directed toward measuring the value of quality. This effort would require, first, the determination of which qualities or styles of care produce improvements in outcomes, and, second, a method for valuing those improvements according to some common standard. The standard should not be limited to a narrow definition of "health," but should include the social and psychological aspects of care as well. These estimates could then assist policymakers in determining the appropriate social budget for health care and could be used to provide information to consumers on the consequences of their choices. In addition, further evaluation of the results of PSROs, utilization review, and second opinion surgical programs should be encouraged to determine their contribution to improved quality.

Information

The fourth principal cause of hospital cost inflation is the lack of expertise on the part of consumers in determining an appropriate mix of medical therapies. Physicians, because of expert knowledge, have tended to substitute their judgment for that of the consumer. Two aspects of this situation warrant further investigation. First, PSROs, utilization review, and second opinion surgical programs should be reexamined to determine if their use can be expanded to improve physicians' and consumers' decisionmaking. Second, the lifting of restrictions on the advertising of physician fees, hospital charges, drug prices, and the prices of medical devices should be considered. Such changes are particularly important if indemnity insurance is introduced, since consumers would then be required to choose among providers on the basis of cost as well as quality. In particular, insurance arrangements that encourage insurers to introduce cost control efforts by permitting them to offer lower premiums when those efforts succeed should be encouraged. The tax treatment of employer-paid health insurance premiums, which encourages expensive first-dollar coverage, should be reviewed.

Competition as a Cost Control Strategy

The usual approach to cost control is to induce competition that provides incentives for cost reduction via the price mechanism. In the health care sector, competition can be provided through HMOs and alternative insurance arrangements. Present federal policy provides no incentives for Medicare and Medicaid eligibles to choose lower cost providers because there is no reward for such a choice. Permitting such persons to share part of the cost savings from choosing more efficient providers in the form of expanded benefits would seem to be desirable.

In a more general sense, competition among HMOs and alternative insurance plans may help to control costs. In particular, it may be possible for insurers to develop effective cost and utilization control strategies and to permit consumers to choose among those strategies on the basis of relative premiums and benefits.

Part II

Background Document

INTRODUCTION

The administration's Hospital Cost Containment Act of 1977 (HR 6575) and Senator Talmadge's Medicare—Medicaid Administration and Reimbursement Reform Act (S 1470) are largely responses to the rapidly rising cost of health care. The analysis here will provide both a statement of the dimensions of the health care inflation problem and a critical examination of the mechanisms and procedures that have been used in an attempt to stem the rate of inflation. Using this analysis as background, the anticipated effectiveness of the two cost containment proposals are assessed in terms of both their effects on hospital costs and their effects on the nature, delivery, and quality of health care services. The proposals will be evaluated in terms of a set of short-term and long-term objectives that we believe any effective cost containment program should strive for. These objectives are:

1. *To be consistent with a National Health Insurance (NHI) program.* The analysis provided here will neither assess the desirability of NHI nor evaluate alternative designs for such a program. It will, however, assess the effectiveness of the proposed cost containment programs in reducing the rate of increase in health care costs.
2. *To reduce the level of inefficiency in the health care system, for example, by reducing the number of underused beds and avoiding the duplication of services.*

3. *To alter the decisionmaking mechanisms and organization of the industry, to restructure incentives, and to alter the goals of providers in order to provide health care services that are appropriate at a reasonable cost.* While hospitals account for the largest single share of health care expenditures, effects on other providers indirectly affected by the legislation must also be considered.

4. *To permit learning from experience with a specific program so that it can be revised, improved, or possibly eliminated in light of that experience.* A cost containment plan should be adaptive and adaptable, so that performance can be used to guide future adjustments. The administration proposes a "purely transitional program" intended to give the nation a breather from the rapid increase in health care costs until the unveiling of a longer range cost containment program that would be fully effective in the early 1980s. The objective of "experiential learning" is clearly a very important criterion in evaluating both the administration and the Talmadge proposals.

5. *To apply cost containment controls in a manner that offers a realistic likelihood for achieving results and to apply the controls to those components of the system most likely to yield cost savings.* Controls can be applied to the operating costs and/or capital expenditures of providers or to the revenue received by providers. An advantage of revenue control is that it creates an incentive for the administrator of a hospital to use his best judgment in determining how to control costs. An advantage of expenditure control is that it permits more direct alteration of the outcome of the resource allocation process. In addition to the nature of the mechanisms used to alter the rate of cost increase, a program must deal with the issue of the target of these mechanisms. For example, the controls in the administration's proposal apply only to inpatient revenue, while the Talmadge proposal covers outpatient costs but exempts certain classes of costs. The appropriate breadth of coverage will be a concern of this analysis.

6. *To apply cost containment controls in as equitable a manner as possible.*

7. *To be consistent with and encourage more fundamental reforms in insurance, organization, and reimbursement arrangements, which may at some future date make direct cost controls unnecessary.*

Chapter 3

The Cost Containment Problem: Scope, Causes, and Attempts at Resolution

HOSPITAL COST INFLATION

Table 3—1 indicates the rate of increase in selected hospital cost indicators in recent years. Most of the data refer to cost per adjusted admission, insofar as admissions is the unit of output or volume to be used in the administration's proposed cost containment program. The first part of the table presents monetary increases in nominal terms, while the second part adjusts those increases for the effects of general inflation. The rates in the second part of the table therefore reflect the rates of increase in hospital costs in constant dollars or the rates of increase in the relative price of hospital care.

It is possible to distinguish several periods in the data. First, there was a substantial surge in the rate of inflation following the passage of Medicare and Medicaid in 1966. This rate was beginning to taper off, especially in real terms, when the Economic Stabilization Program (ESP) was begun in late 1971. ESP will be discussed in more detail in a later section, but it can be seen here that it produced a significant drop in the nominal rate of inflation, only to be followed by a return up to and beyond the prior rate when the controls were lifted in 1974. The real rate of inflation, however, was equally affected by ESP. It actually continued to decline for a while after the program was terminated. Both real and nominal costs increased at a rapid rate in 1975 and 1976.

The table also indicates that the inflation was composed of both increases in prices for hospital inputs (measured by wages per employee and the American Hospital Association's nonlabor input price index) and increases in inputs, labor and nonlabor, per adjusted pa-

Table 3–1.   Annual Rates of Increase, Selected Hospital Time Series.

Year	Expenses per Adjusted Admission	Expenses per Adjusted Inpatient Day	Nominal Terms				Nonlabor Inputs per Admission	Length of Stay
			Total Expenses	FTE Personnel per Adjusted Admission	Labor Earnings per FTE Personnel	Nonlabor Input Price (all items)		
	a	a	a	a	a	b	ab	a
1963			10.1		3.7			1.3
1964	8.2	7.0	10.8	2.2	6.0			0.0
1965	8.2	7.9	9.6	4.3	5.4			1.3
1966	10.6	7.6	12.3	8.3	0.7			1.3
1967	17.6	13.3	17.6	5.8	9.3			5.1
1968	15.3	12.8	17.2	3.6	9.8	3.6	13.0	1.2
1969	14.5	15.2	17.3	3.5	9.3	4.3	12.0	-1.2
1970	12.8	14.7	17.7	1.7	10.0	5.5	9.0	-1.2
1971	10.3	13.2	14.5	0.0	10.3	4.2	6.5	-2.4
1972	11.1	13.4	14.1	0.0	8.1	4.0	11.0	-1.2
1973	6.7	7.6	11.5	0.0	4.5	8.3	1.3	-1.3
1974	10.5	11.2	14.9	1.7	5.7	17.4*	-4.1	0.0
1975	16.6	17.6	19.4	3.3	10.9	20.8*	-.05	-1.3
1976	13.2	13.7	15.4	1.6	8.1	10.1**	6.9	0.0
1977								

*Figures may be misleading. AHA is currently revising the index for these periods.
**3rd quarter 1976—3rd quarter 1977.

Table 3–1. continued

Year	Nominal Terms (cont'd.)				Real Terms		
	Consumer Price Index (less medical care)	Hospital Cost Index	Hospital Intensity Index	Net Total Revenue per Adjusted Admission	Expenses per Adjusted Admission	Expenses per Adjusted Patient Day	Net Revenue per Adjusted Admission
	c	b	b	a			
1963	1.2						
1964	1.3				6.9	5.7	
1965	1.5				6.7	6.4	
1966	2.9				7.7	4.7	
1967	2.4				15.2	10.9	
1968	4.1				11.2	8.7	
1969	5.4				9.1	9.8	
1970	5.8	8.7	9.6		7.0	8.9	
1971	4.1	6.3	5.3		6.2	9.1	
1972	3.3	3.4	3.2	9.8	7.8	10.1	6.5
1973	6.4	4.9	1.8	5.9	0.3	1.2	−0.5
1974	11.1	9.2	4.0	10.6	−0.6	0.1	−0.5
1975	8.9	11.9	4.6	16.5	7.7	8.7	7.6
1976	5.5	10.0	5.5	15.5	7.7	8.2	10.0
1977		9.4	4.7				

Sources:

a: Hospital Statistics, American Hospital Association, Annual Surveys 1965–1976.
b: American Hospital Association.
c: *Social Security Bulletin*, DHEW, April 1977.

tient day or per adjusted admission. Indeed, Feldstein and Taylor have shown that this increase in "intensity" of care accounted for about three-fourths of the real increase in cost per adjusted patient day during the period.[1] That is, if hospital input prices had increased at the same rate as prices generally, real increases in price would have been only 25 percent less. Increases in intensity were less important in explaining the increase in cost per adjusted admission, in part because of a decline in length of stay. When the American Hospital Association's nonlabor input price index is used to calculate nonlabor inputs per adjusted admission, there is some suggestion that the rate of increase in input intensity began to slacken in 1974–1975, although the results may be affected by the erratic behavior of that index. Perhaps the effects of the increase in third party coverage in the 1960s finally began to wear off. The hospital intensity index, which was developed by the American Hospital Association to track the quantities of services per adjusted patient day, has also increased less rapidly in 1977 than in 1976. Most of the cost increases in these years appears to have resulted from increases in hospital input costs, especially for malpractice insurance and energy.

IMPORTANCE OF THE PROBLEM

The fundamental health care problem addressed in this analysis is the rise in the relative price of health care services. The real problem is not the "contribution" of health care inflation to overall inflation, but rather the increase in real inputs, both per unit of output and in total, devoted to the health care sector. The nation is expending an increasing share of its resources on health, and the public and policymakers have begun to ask whether the nation is receiving appreciable improvements in health status or well-being for this increased expenditure.

The rapid rate of hospital cost inflation has had adverse consequences on several parts of the economy. It has reduced what consumers have left to spend on other goods they value. The 50 percent increase in the share of gross national product going to health care since 1960 has meant that consumers have had to sacrifice more and more, both proportionately and in total, for the health care they have received. What they have had to pay out of pocket at the point of service has not increased much in real terms and for some types of care (e.g., hospital care) has actually declined because of broader insurance coverage. However, these reductions have resulted in offsetting increases in health insurance premiums and in taxes needed to pay for the care received. Surveys of consumer attitudes indicate that, while consumers are generally satisfied with the health care they receive, they would prefer that it be less expensive. While the current rate of increase in health care expenditures could well continue for some time, it cannot do so forever. At present, each worker must work the equivalent of one month a year to pay for health care, and this is up from about two and one half weeks a generation ago. The critical question is whether our citizenry is getting sufficient value for this effort.

The rapid increases in costs have caused difficulty for third party payers as well as for consumers. Private insurance companies have in the recent past run underwriting losses because of their inability to correctly anticipate cost increases. They presently show no disposition to abandon the health insurance business, however, since they are able to keep premiums rising in line with benefits. More serious than the effect on private insurance companies has been the effect of inflation on the federal and state governments providing health insurance or health care. Extreme underestimates of program costs for Medicare and Medicaid induced both the federal and state governments to offer more extensive and comprehensive programs than they would have done had they correctly anticipated the true costs. The result of the increased costs has been de facto program cutbacks and reductions in benefits, combined with financial distress for some states because of their Medicaid programs. Planners failed to take account of the rapid rate of price increase in health care caused by the Medicare and Medicaid programs themselves. Thus, the increased expenditures have caused a displacement not just of private spending but of public spending as well. Had inflation been more controlled, there might well have been larger expenditures for mental health, consumer education, housing, environmental protection, and sanitation—programs that could have a substantial impact on health.

A third effect of increased expenditures has been a redistribution of income from consumers of health care to suppliers of specialized factor inputs, such as health care professionals and firms producing medical supplies. The redistribution to hospital-based health professionals has also been pronounced, as will be shown elsewhere in this document. While hospital workers as a whole still have low incomes relative to all workers, their incomes are not low relative to those of other workers of comparable skill level. In particular, registered nurses have made substantial gains in recent years and earn wages in excess of those of similar skill levels in other employment situations.[2]

Finally, it has been alleged that inflation has delayed the introduction of some form of national health insurance (NHI). This is a political rather than an economic welfare argument. From a purely theoretical viewpoint, the increased insurance coverage embodied in most NHI schemes would actually be more valuable the higher the hospital costs. From a political viewpoint, however, regardless of the validity of the above observation, it may not be prudent in a period of large federal deficits to embark on a program that would not only be costly now but would also be likely to be a drain on the federal budget in the future.

THE CAUSES OF THE PROBLEM OF RISING HOSPITAL COSTS AND EXPENDITURES

This section will analyze the problem of hospital cost inflation without explicit treatment of possible changes in the quality or style of hospital care. Those issues involved in measuring and evaluating such changes will be discussed in the following section.

Introduction

The hospital cost problem is the result of a multiplicity of factors. These factors lead the hospital care "market" to function inefficiently in the sense that, at the margin, the value of hospital care to consumers is not as great as the value of the goods they must sacrifice in order to pay the cost of the provision of that care. This inefficiency is reflected both in the burden that hospital costs place on individual consumers, primarily in the form of insurance premiums, and in the burden placed on the public sector in the allocation of its budgets.

The failure of the market to function effectively is due to both demand and supply effects. The demand effects are largely the result of widespread insurance coverage that has reduced the price of care to a small fraction of its cost. The supply effects are caused both by the desire of providers to render improved quality almost without regard to cost and by the proliferation of cost-increasing technological innovations. These two effects are discussed below.

Demand

Insurance. The predominant form of hospital insurance pays benefits that increase with increases in expenditures for hospital care. With most forms of insurance coverage, once the insurance premium is paid, the patient incurs no further, or almost no further, out of pocket costs regardless of whether he consumes more units of hospital care or more costly styles of the same care. Thus, since both the patient and the physician usually prefer more care to less, and since higher quality is preferred to lower quality, patients and/or their physicians can be expected to demand more costly forms of care when a patient has insurance than when he does not. In effect, insurance reduces the user price of care below its market price and below its true cost. This leads to additional quantities being consumed—for example, more frequent hospitalization or higher surgical rates. It also leads to greater cost per unit, as qualitatively better and more expensive units of care are provided. Consumers will indirectly bear some of this cost through higher insurance premiums, but even that effect is often obscured by employer contributions to insurance premiums.

Preferences of Providers. Coupled with the effect of insurance coverage is the inability and/or unwillingness of health care providers to deal with the issue of the "value" of improvements in medical care. Tradeoffs between the quality of health care and the cost of providing that care are made only reluctantly, and thus little pressure is exerted in opposition to proposed increases in the quality of care, however costly. The reduced direct cost to patients because of insurance coverage and the unwillingness of decisionmakers to make cost-quality decisions result in little pressure for expenditure control.

In many markets, downward pressure on prices is exercised by large purchasers of an industry's product. In health care, Blue Cross, Blue Shield, and the private insurers might have been expected to exert a control over cost, but there is little evidence that they have chosen to play this role. Certainly, till recently they have not played a major part in effective efforts to hold down the rate of cost increases. Whether the efforts under the current voluntary effort will be successful is discussed in Appendix C.

Supply

Objectives of Providers. On the supply side, one of the peculiar characteristics of the health care industry is that nearly all the providers may have objectives of higher priority than cost minimization. The specific goals of these providers are open to debate, but most observers would agree that hospital trustees, administrators, and affiliated physicians count among their objectives the provision of modern facilities, the provision of high quality and comprehensive services, efficiency, and appropriate rewards for employees and physician staffs. To meet these goals, a hospital must set its priorities. One plausible premise is that hospitals strive to achieve all of these objectives to varying extents. Since hospitals know that, because of insurance coverage, the high cost associated with additional services will not be directly borne by the consumer and that third party payers can be reasonably expected to reimburse them for the incurred costs, they have the opportunity to pursue their goals with little economic risk in their decisions. This is not to argue that hospitals desire to be wasteful or inefficient, but instead that they seek to expand services. A motivation for expansion is undoubtedly the desire to provide higher quality care to the community served by the hospital. In addition, their administrators and physicians attain status and satisfaction from being associated with a modern, well-equipped hospital.

These objectives provide a continuing pressure for increased expenditures both for equipment and facilities and for additional personnel. For example, Dr. Edgar T. Beddingfield, Jr., then a practicing physician and chairman of the Council on Legislation of the American Medical Association, stated in testimony on HR 6575 before the joint hearings of the House Subcommittee on Health, Committee on Ways and Means, and the House Subcommittee on Health and the Environment, Committee on Interstate and Foreign Commerce, on May 13, 1977:

> In order to provide an uninterrupted flow of quality hospital care which the American people demand, a hospital must keep pace with current technological advances. This often means purchase of expensive equipment. This often also means the necessity to expand services. No patient wishes to be admitted to a hospital which he believes is not a modern hospital. . . .[3]

A similar theme was stressed in the testimony of the Association of American Medical Colleges to the same subcommittees:

> As a public resource, hospitals are expected to meet the needs of their community. Therefore, hospitals have added new services, equipment, and personnel to meet the public's desire for access to the latest medical and scientific accomplishments.[4]

While a hospital's net revenue or profit is typically used to extend services and to provide modern equipment, it may also indirectly increase the returns to providers such as physicians. Physicians may wish a hospital to expand its facilities or to use its services more intensively in the care of patients because their own productivity, and accordingly, income could be increased.

If a physician's patient had extensive insurance coverage and desired a wide range of expensive services, the physician would most likely want the hospital to provide those services. Not to do so would mean that the physician was not acting in the patient's best interest.

Support for the role of the physician in influencing the services provided to patients can be found in the testimony of John F. Horty, president of the National Council of Community Hospitals, on HR 6575 to the same Subcommittees on Health:

> Only physicians have the authority to admit and discharge patients, and to determine the intensity and mix of medical treatment. What sort of patient is hospitalized, how many tests are given, and what sort of overall care is accorded are matters currently within the sole prerogative of the physician, who in large part makes these determinations free from hospital control or influence and without the need to consider economic factors.[5]

With the principal decisionmakers for the utilization of medical services holding the objectives expressed above and with such diminished incentives for cost containment facing them, there is little reason to expect that either hospitals or physicians would enter into discussions of whether the benefits from improvements in health care resulting from the pursuit of quality goals are worth the cost.

Rising Wage Rates. A further cause of hospital inflation has been the rising wage rates of hospital employees. Improving the wages of employees, even at a cost to consumers and third party payers, has been high priority for hospital administrators in recent years. Indeed, there is some evidence to suggest that hospitals may have philanthropic wage policies toward their employees. It will be shown later that the wages paid to hospital employees have tended to catch up to, and in some cases to surpass, those in the private sector for certain occupational classes.

Technological Change. Another cause of hospital cost inflation relates to the supply of medical technology available to hospitals. A report by the Council on Wage and Price Stability states:

> New technology in medicine, unlike that in other industries, has unfortunately tended, on the whole, to be cost-raising rather than cost-reducing.[6]

Similarly, the Association of American Medical Colleges, in their testimony on the administration's proposal, attributes inflation in part to changes in the style and sophistication of care and equipment.[7]

An effect of broad and comprehensive insurance coverage and of an unwillingness to make cost-quality tradeoffs is the tendency of individuals and their physicians to elect almost any service or treatment that might improve the patient's health or well-being. At any given time, the number of regimens that can be effectively applied to a given patient is necessarily limited. Over time, if providers are confident that they can generate the revenue needed to cover the cost of new technology, the number of possibly beneficial devices or procedures that could be developed and marketed would appear to be quite large. There may also be a "technological imperative" operating in the sense that new devices, once generated, tend to be adopted.[8] It should therefore not be surprising that technological change in hospitals can be rapid and expensive. The primary causes of this technological change, however, would appear to be the insurance coverage, which has paid the bill for the introduction of expensive technology; reimbursement mechanisms that do not provide a check on cost increases; and provider desire to improve the quality of care.

Other Special Characteristics.   There are other special characteristics of the health care market that combine with insurance coverage to distort the market further. One characteristic is that information about prices or qualities of different therapeutic options is difficult to obtain. Professional codes and state laws typically prohibit the dissemination of price information, and consumers are sometimes unable to assess quality differences.

In addition, insurance coverage reduces consumers' incentives to search for lower prices. If there were a difference in price and cost between two hospitals, the consumer will surely be less motivated to find out which hospital is less expensive when his insurance pays the full charge of either hospital. Consequently, insurance not only persuades consumers to use more, as well as higher quality and more expensive, care, it also reduces the extent to which providers have to compete.

Inefficiency and the Supply of Care

One common assertion regarding hospital performance is that hospitals are inefficient in the provision of their services. It does not seem reasonable, however, to argue that hospitals are inefficient in what could be termed a "technical" sense. That is, it is doubtful that, on average, a hospital could produce the same output it is currently producing, at the same quality (however defined), with substantially fewer inputs. There is no conclusive evidence to support the proposition that there is "slack" in the production process of an appreciable number of individual hospitals, in the sense that each hospital is not producing its product at minimum cost. Most of the observed differences across hospitals in costs per patient day or per admission can be accounted for either by differences in the prices they pay for inputs, by characteristics of output such as case mix, or by input intensity.[9] Hospitals are not, in general, inefficiently run firms, and hospital administrations ought not to be criticized on this score.

If there are inefficiencies in the provision of hospital services, these inefficiencies are of two other types. One might be called "system inefficiency"—that is, higher than necessary costs for the total output of a given quality produced by the hospital system caused by the way the system (rather than any individual hospital) is organized. The other type of inefficiency could be termed cost-quality inefficiency. This second kind of inefficiency occurs when cost increases are accompanied by quality increases, but the value of these quality increases falls short of the costs needed to produce them. Both of these types of inefficiency have contributed to hospital cost inflation.

System inefficiency generally occurs when the inputs needed to produce some kind of output come in fixed or indivisible amounts and when there are problems in the distribution of that output across hospitals. For example, the volume of cases handled by an open heart surgery unit needs to be of some minimum size in order for that unit to be efficiently utilized. Suppose that, because of the presence of open heart surgery units in many hospitals in a given area, none of the units is able to operate at sufficient capacity to be efficient. The costs of their collective output could be lowered by concentrating such units in a smaller number of hospitals, thus lowering capital and operating expenditures. As new services and equipment are introduced, excessive systemwide expansion of services can contribute to increasing costs and to a higher rate of inflation. This kind of system inefficiency would appear to pose a problem for the U.S. hospital system and is encouraged by the cost-based reimbursement nature of much of hospital insurance.

Cost-quality inefficiency is a less obvious, but important, contributor to rising costs. Higher levels of quality of hospital care, whether measured by the modernity of buildings and equipment, the availability of specialized facilities, the breadth of services offered, or the guarantee that an emergency patient will find a bed, are valued by hospitals, physicians, and patients. The critical point is that this value should not be sought at any price. At some point, the cost of a reduction in the probability that a bed will be unavailable, the cost of an additional diagnostic test, or the cost of the convenience to a patient of having a special facility available in a given hospital rather that his (her) having to be transported to another may reach a level that exceeds the benefit derived.

The goal of an effective health care system should be the provision of an appropriate level of quality—namely, that level at which the benefits from additional quality just cover its additional costs. It is possible to have too much of a good thing—too much in the sense that quality can cost too much in terms of other good things foregone. In the case of hospital care, these other things could be more accessible ambulatory care, more preventive medicine, better nutrition, better housing, or other goods that people value. There is good reason to believe that current levels of hospital quality may be higher than appropriate and that the cost of this quality has accounted for much of the recent hospital cost inflation. As noted above, under present forms of hospitalization insurance, neither the consumer nor his physician needs to consider much, if any, of the cost of extra quality, because that cost is covered by insurance, public or private.

Much of the recent increase in hospital costs arises from higher levels of inputs, both personnel and equipment, per patient day or per admission. Feldstein and Taylor estimate that three-fourths of the recent rise in hospital cost per patient day relative to the general price level has been due to increased volume of such inputs.[10] The inputs are not worthless; the critical question, however, is whether they are worth the increased costs.

The fundamental issue that will eventually have to be faced is which quality improvements, if any, will have to be foregone because their cost is judged to be too great. Individual hospitals have not, in the past, faced this question because the incentives facing them did not induce them to do so. No purpose is served in finding fault with past decisions of hospitals, when they were responding appropriately to the incentives with which society presented them. In addition, it is not obvious that individual hospitals can make these cost-quality tradeoffs appropriately or that they should make them. Policymakers will have to perform at least part of this distasteful task. Rather than blaming hospitals, it would seem more worthwhile for federal policymakers to commit resources to begin both developing the mechanisms necessary to make such decisions rationally and explaining to voters the need for such decisions.

ISSUES IN THE ASSESSMENT OF QUALITY OF CARE

Of the issues entailed in an analysis of hospital cost containment, one of the most perplexing is that of assessing the nature of the change in quality of care, if any, associated with the increased hospital costs. Two basic questions derive from this concern: (1) have the increased labor and nonlabor inputs into a unit of hospital care resulted in an increase in the quality of that care, and (2) if such a quality increase has occurred, has it been worth the social cost of the resources needed to produce it? Apologists for the current trends in hospital costs allege an increase in the quality of hospital care. Critics of the hospital industry, however, are quick to dismiss the possibility that such quality changes have indeed altered the nature of the hospital care received and that an improved product is now being produced. The problem is compounded by the difficulty of incorporating a measure of quality of care into the various measures of hospital output. This difficulty most often results both in quality dimensions not being included in such output measures and in an implicit judgment therein that quality has not changed.

Central to the problem of attempting to incorporate quality dimensions into measures of a hospital's product are the problems both of specifying an appropriate definition of what constitutes "quality" care and of finding indexes suitably sensitive to measure changes in that quality. Students of the art of quality assessment have identified three types of variables for evaluating the quality of medical care: structure, process, and outcome variables. The first of these assesses the characteristics of the providers of care; the second, the specific items of the care delivered; and the third, the changes in the physical and/or psychological state of the patient, if any, as a result of the care received. Examples of structural variables include the teaching versus nonteaching status of hospitals, the nature of the training of physicians (foreign versus U.S. graduates), and the certification status of surgeons. Studies utilizing structural variables have suggested that higher levels of care (defined mostly by process measures internal to each study) are, in certain instances, associated with certain structural characteristics.[11] Such studies, however, are far from conclusive in establishing as clear-cut an association of certain structural characteristics with superior care as the "conventional wisdom" would often have us believe.[12]

Assessment of the process of care entails a judgment of the appropriateness of the presence/absence, frequency/dose, and so forth, of a specific event (e.g., test, drug, etc.) in the care of a patient. The appropriateness of the event can be assessed either in terms of the implicit judgment of a physician or other individual reviewing the case or in terms of standards explicitly formulated by physicians as to what constitutes quality care in such a case.[13] Studies have found deficiencies in the process of care that range from modest to severe.[14] Care is generally rated higher in studies utilizing implicit criteria than in those utilizing explicit criteria. Such variability in the assessment of the process of care has raised serious questions as to the ultimate utility of this mode of assessment.[15] The utility of process assessment is further compromised insofar as little is known about the sensitivity of the outcome of care to the individual process items. Indeed, studies have shown that acceptable outcomes can follow from allegedly poor process.[16] This gap in knowledge is especially critical to the issue of increased hospital costs. If the increase in the inputs into hospital care has not resulted in improved outcomes, one can legitimately argue that only the "style" of care, not the "quality," has changed and that a true inflation in costs has occurred. If, on the other hand, the increased inputs were associated with bona fide improvements in outcomes, we would not be dealing with inflation per se but the increased cost of an improved product.

This problem of attempting to determine aggregate outcome changes is exacerbated by the problem of finding vital statistics or indexes sensitive enough to reflect aggregate changes in the quality of hospital care. Scant attention has been paid to investigating whether the increased inputs into hospital care have resulted in increased quality. For instance, in documenting the increased inputs per unit of hospital service in his study, "The Rising Cost of Hospital Care," Feldstein is very careful not to speculate whether quality changes have resulted.[17] While not addressing this issue as its primary focus, the work of Scitovsky and McCall does, however, shed some suggestive light on it.[18] Scitovsky and McCall investigated the magnitude of the changes in hospital costs in one hospital setting due to changes in inputs to care for small groups of patients in eight diagnostic categories over the period of the early 1950s, the mid-1960s, and the early 1970s. They noted that, with the exception of decreased length of stay for most of the diagnostic categories, inputs into care in most of the categories had increased. Though they based the bulk of their discussion on current dollar estimates, they noted that these input changes were on balance cost raising.

Of particular note were the increased inputs into the care of appendicitis (simple and perforated) and myocardial infarction. In the case of appendicitis, they noted that, for the period 1951–1964, "the main factors that raised costs for both types of appendicitis were: an increase in the number of laboratory tests per case (from 4.7 to 7.3 for simple appendicitis, from 5.3 to 14.5 for perforated), an increase in the average number of postoperative intravenous solutions (from 0.1 to 2.4 for simple appendicitis, from 6.7 to 12.7 for perforated appendicitis). . . ."[19] Though the magnitude of the relative increase was slightly reduced in the period 1964–1971, similar trends were also noted then.

In the case of acute myocardial infarction, they noted a substantial increase of the input "intensive coronary care" over the period 1964–1971 as well as substantial increases in the number of EKGs, X-rays, and laboratory tests ordered and in the amount of intravenous and inhalation therapy employed. They calculated that these input changes accounted for 33 percent of the increase in the cost of treatment of myocardial infarction from 1964 to 1971 and, using current dollar values and national data on the prevalence of myocardial infarction, estimated that these input changes could have accounted nationally for as much as $275 million of the additional health expenditures in 1971 as compared to 1964.

After presenting these data, Scitovsky and McCall devote the thrust of their discussion to arguing against the absolutist and simplistic "more is better" school without seeming to raise the question as to whether some of the "more" inputs might not be better. This increase in the number of tests in appendicitis could conceivably have been, in the preoperative phase, a response of surgeons attempting to reduce the number of "unnecessary" appendectomies and accordingly could have prevented some operations. Similarly, in the case of appendicitis, an interesting question arises as to whether the increased use of postoperative intravenous solutions could have been associated with diminished postoperative gastrointestinal complications and hence a contributor to the decreased length of stay noted by the authors.

The precise relationship of such process items to improved outcomes in appendicitis is questioned, however, by the provocative study of Fessel and Van Brunt.[20] They investigated the differences in the process of care of acute appendicitis in a university hospital and a nonuniversity hospital and attempted to correlate the observed process differences with outcome differences. Needless to say, the community hospital setting scored much lower on the number of tests performed and so forth and would have received bad grades on any process scores. Investigation of the outcomes of care between the two settings (in terms of complication rates, etc.) showed no differences, however. The results of Fessel and Van Brunt's study suggest that much of the differential process of medical care in the university setting compared to the community hospital was not contributing to quality differences per se (as measured in the study) and might legitimately be labeled "style" differences. This contention might also apply to Scitovsky and McCall's findings insofar as, over the periods of their study, the hospital under study was progressively increasing the scope of its educational programs and evolving into a major university teaching hospital. This point is not articulated by

Scitovsky and McCall, but it is reasonable to believe that some of the input changes noted by them were an outgrowth of a change of style in the hospital encompassing a greater teaching emphasis.

The case for substantial outcome changes being associated with the increased inputs into the care of myocardial infarction is a much stronger one, however. After presenting their data on these increased inputs, Scitovsky and McCall cite the fact that the age-adjusted mortality rate from myocardial infarction in the United States fell from 141.1 for 100,000 in 1968 to 127.0 in 1971—a decrease of almost 10 percent in three years. They proceed, however, to cite literature questioning the efficacy of coronary care units and do not seriously address the possibility that such increased inputs over the United States as a whole could be responsible for the decrease in mortality. In testimony before the Senate Health Subcommittee of the Health and Scientific Research Committee on Human Resources, Dorothy Rice, Director of the National Center for Health Statistics, was more positive. In noting the decline in deaths from heart disease she stated:

> The decline in heart disease deaths may reflect better medical care, since surveys on hospital discharges show that the rate of incidence of heart disease has not fallen although the death rate for the disease has dropped.[21]

The aggregate vital statistics of the United States and their relative stability in the recent past are frequently used to question the quality of the medical care in the United States and to argue against the possibility of quality improvements resulting from increased inputs. In 1976, the United States recorded its lowest age-adjusted death rate, its lowest infant mortality rate, and its lowest maternal mortality rate, while age-specific death rates from heart disease continued to fall.[22] In view of the continued and sustained improvement in these indexes, it would appear appropriate that the question of the extent to which input changes in the United States health system may be expressing themselves in improved health status of the population be reopened and systematically investigated. The possibility of an improved health status as a function of increased inputs into our medical care is a critical question in the current policy debate on hospital cost containment. Pending empirical validation of an increased input-improved health outcome causality, one would hope that flexibility would be maintained in any cost containment policy promulgated so that efficacious quality improvements could be further developed and disseminated while "pure style" changes were discouraged.

An additional and important question that must be addressed in evaluating the "value" of the increased inputs into medical care process is the extent to which they generate a sense of well-being in the consumer that extends beyond pure physical gain and entails such benefits as reduced anxiety, reassurance, and knowledge that one is receiving a "proper" process of medical care. This sense of well-being can be a commodity that is being purchased along with the medical care itself. It is valued highly by most clinicians and described by Fuchs as an integral component of a successful medical care transaction.[23] This sense of well-being is most often not even acknowledged, let alone quantified, in attempts to measure the value of medical care received. It would appear reasonable that the value to the consumer of this "sense of well-being" would increase in proportion to the magnitude of the threat of his illness to survival.

Even if a causation between increased process inputs and improved health outcomes were to be demonstrated, the critical question, as discussed above, is whether the improved health outcomes warrant the social costs involved. A recent study by Cullen et al. speaks to this question.[24] Cullen et al. measured the charges that accrued to a population of 226 consecutive critically ill patients who required intensive care following surgery and investigated the survival rate of these patients at selected time intervals up to one year following hospitalization. An articulated rationale for the study was that "physicians responsible for ordering health care expect unlimited resources to be marshalled for the critically ill patient and yet remain unaware of the results of their efforts."[25] The average charge for the hospitalization of the 226 patients was $14,304. After one month, 123 (54 percent) of the patients were dead. At twelve months, 164, or almost three-quarters, of the patients were dead; 11 were still hospitalized, and 51 were at home. Only twenty-six of the sixty-two survivors had fully recovered. To all intents and purposes, the intensive care used to treat these patients did not exist twenty years ago. In this series of cases, it undoubtedly produced some transiently improved and, quite possibly, some permanently improved outcomes compared to what might have been possible at that time. The question remains, however, of the size of benefits that could accrue from alternative forms of investments of the resources used in the intensive care of these patients.

The question of the relationship of increased inputs into hospital care to quality changes is thus a complex one. It is done justice neither by those who, in addressing the problem of the rise in the cost of hospitalization, axiomatically claim "more is better" nor by those who appear to categorically ignore the possibility that quality has improved.[26]

THE CONTRIBUTION OF DEMOGRAPHIC CHANGES TO HOSPITAL COSTS AND EXPENDITURES

Throughout the period of rising hospital costs, the demographic characteristics of the population have been changing. In particular, there have been increases in the proportion of people over sixty-five years of age and a decrease in the proportion of children. The proportion of the population over sixty-five years of age increased from 9.6 percent in 1966 to about 10.4 percent in 1975. People over sixty-five have more frequent episodes of hospitalization than the general population. On average, these episodes tend to last longer and to be more costly. For example, the mean length of stay for persons discharged from hospitals subscribing to the PAS information system is about 90 percent greater for persons over sixty-five than for those under sixty-five (omitting newborns).[27] The mean hospital cost per capita for the population over sixty-five was 3.1 times greater than the mean cost for the entire population in fiscal 1974. If the same ratio of relative expenditures prevailed over the past ten years, demographic change would have accounted for an increase in per capita real hospital expenditures over the entire period of about 2.5 percent or 0.25 percent per year. While the expenditures suggested by these figures are not insubstantial in absolute dollars, they do suggest that the increase in age has not been a principal contributor to the increase in hospital costs per capita.

HMOs AND HOSPITAL COSTS

One of the mechanisms suggested for controlling high health care costs is the spread of health maintenance organizations (HMOs) or prepaid group practices. The major cost advantage of the HMO over conventional forms of insurance and practice organization stems from the lower rates of hospital admissions in HMOs. Interestingly, costs per patient day or per hospital episode are about the same in HMOs as in the conventional system.

There are two ways in which the spread of HMO-type arrangements might reduce hospital costs. First, increased participation in HMOs may lower hospital costs for subscribing members. Second, customary providers of medical care may hold their costs down in order not to be at a competitive disadvantage relative to HMOs. While HMO hospital costs per enrollee are about 20–25 percent lower than under conventional insurance, the rate of increase in these costs has not been substantially lower than that in the conventional sector.[28] All other things being equal, a substantial shift from conventional insurance to HMOs could thus have a significant effect on hospital costs, but it may be only a "one shot" effect.

Moreover, even if the one shot effect were large in absolute terms, it is unlikely to have a substantial effect on the rate of cost increase. For example, suppose that, by dint of herculean effort, half of the U.S. population could be enrolled in HMOs over the next ten years and that an average saving of 20 percent of hospital expenditures per enrollee could be achieved. Such an effort would reduce the inflation rate by only 1 percent per year.

Definitive evidence on the inflation rate for HMOs is not available. Comparison of rates of change in cost per enrollee or cost per unit of output between HMO and non–HMO members is difficult because of the changing age–sex composition of each group of subscribers and because of increases in the benefits provided by non–HMO insurance policies. Preliminary results of a study by Luft suggest that HMOs have had a lower inflation rate, but that the difference between it and that in the conventional sector has been slight.[29]

The short-run effect on non–HMO hospital costs of a substantial shift to HMOs would probably be to raise expenditures per unit of hospital care in the non–HMO sector. Even though a reduction in non–HMO hospital use in the short run would reduce total costs somewhat, the unit cost would rise, as overhead costs would have to be spread over fewer admissions. In the long run, however, with an appropriate closing or transfer of facilities, the net effect of HMOs could be to reduce both unit and total costs in both sectors.

It is possible that the mere presence of HMOs could keep inflation down, because this presence would create pressures on non–HMO providers to control costs. That is, in states where HMOs are present, other providers may try to reduce their rate of cost inflation in order to stay competitive. Definitive empirical support for this proposition is difficult to obtain because HMO market penetration is significant only in the Western United States where other influences confound the effect of HMOs.

On balance, then, despite the potentially favorable influence of HMOs on costs, it does not appear that competition by HMOs can be relied upon in the short run to correct the hospital cost inflation problem. Strategies to control the present rate of hospital cost increases must concentrate on the existing health delivery system. It is important, however, that the design of a hospital cost containment program not discourage an appropriate spread of HMOs nor undercut efforts by HMOs to improve their competitive positions.

EXPENDITURES ON LONG-TERM CARE

For the last three years, public expenditures for long-term care institutions (LTIs) have constituted a third of Medicaid expenditures. At over $5 billion, they are now greater than the hospital component of Medicaid.[30] For the period 1950–1974, public expenditures for nursing home care grew at an average rate of 28 percent.[31] Federal cost sharing through Medicaid tends to induce state governments to prefer institutional care for the elderly rather than nursing care in housing for the elderly or care provided at home by families, even though such noninstitutional forms of care may be more cost-effective.

Because of Medicaid coverage that reimburses at "reasonable" costs, and possibly because of changes in social attitudes and the demographic structure of the population, LTI occupancy rates have been very high. These high occupancy rates have repeatedly been thought to rationalize approval of new construction. LTI bed availability has been increasing at an average annual rate of 10 percent since 1964.

Some of this growth seems to be a reflection of a housing or custodial function of LTIs. Utilization review required by the 1972 Social Security Act amendments has provided evidence for this viewpoint. It is typically found that a large fraction of the stays of nursing home residents cannot be justified on the basis of medical and nursing needs. For example, in Rhode Island a third or more of residents did not have medical or nursing needs that would justify their presence.[32] The average stay was approximately one year, and very few patients with a stay over one year ever left for home, despite the large fraction capable of living independently with minor attending and supervisory help.

The cost containment proposals analyzed in this volume may have more impact on LTIs, because long-term care can, to some extent, be substituted for acute hospital care. It has been alleged that such substitution would reduce acute hospital costs and total health care expenditures. The average cost per day for hospital inpatient care is several times the average daily cost in a skilled nursing facility. There are, however, some reasons why the actual advantages from substitution may be less than that suggested by average per diem costs. First, when there are unfilled hospital beds, the short-run marginal cost of a day of hospital care can be substantially less than its average cost. In contrast, when LTIs are full, marginal cost is probably at least as great as average cost. Since it is the comparison between marginal costs that is relevant for efficiency, the difference between such costs may be substantially less than that indicated by average costs. Second, one may speculate that extra days of stay in an acute hospital may be socially efficient, even if their cost is greater than that of an equal number of days in an LTI, if the extension of the hospital stay with the provisions of appropriate rehabilitative services can preclude a lengthy stay in an LTI.

The regulation of the LTI industry is too broad a topic for more extensive review in this analysis. If a hospital cost containment program is enacted, however, it may be desirable to modify the admission load formula to encourage a greater reduction in admissions when those admissions are offset by stays in LTIs. The decision to do so should, however, be based on a comparison of actual marginal costs and relative lengths of stay.

THE EXPERIENCE WITH CONTROLS

In this section, several mechanisms and/or attempts to control hospital and health care costs are discussed: prospective reimbursement, certificate of need legislation, the Economic Stabilization Program, Professional Standards Review Organizations, utilization review, second surgical opinion programs, and the Canadian experience with health care budgeting.

Prospective Reimbursement

The central cause of the inflation problem besetting the health industry is a set of institutional arrangements that insulate providers (physicians and hospitals) from market incentives. Prospective reimbursement is designed to deal with this problem of incentives for providers. Additional interest in this mechanism derives from increasing dissatisfaction with the present "open-ended" system of health care financing. Prospective reimbursement represents an attempt at closed-ended funding or "social budgeting" for the hospital component of the health care industry.

The popularity of prospective reimbursement reflects the support it has received from both hospitals and public and private payers. Thomas M. Tierney, former Director of the Bureau of Health Insurance of the Health Care Financing Administration, has observed that hospitals are interested in prospective reimbursement because they believe they will make more money, whereas the government (and other major payers) support prospective reimbursement because they expect to save money.[33]

In early 1976, there were about thirty-five prospective rate-setting systems in operation. Table 3–2 describes the Blue Cross plans with rate setting or review programs, and Table 3–3 describes the hospital rate setting activities of state governments. Prospective reimburse-

Table 3–2.   Blue Cross Plans with Rate Setting or Review Programs as of January 1976.[a]

State or Area Within State	Name of Blue Cross Plan	Number Short-term General and Other Special Hospitals Covered	Percent Plan Area Population Enrolled in Blue Cross
Connecticut	Connecticut Blue Cross	40	51
Indiana	Indiana Blue Cross	115	38
Kentucky	Blue Cross Hospital Plan	107	43
Missouri: Kansas City area	Blue Cross of Kansas City	57	34
New York: New York City	(under state regulation and approvals) Blue Cross–Blue Shield of N.Y.C.	185	73
Upstate	7 upstate plans; as consortium	140	59
North Carolina[b]	Blue Cross and Blue Shield of N.C.	133	34
Ohio: Cincinnati area	Blue Cross of Southwest Ohio	35	59
Oklahoma	Blue Cross and Blue Shield of Oklahoma	40	24
Rhode Island	(with State Office of Budget) Blue Cross of Rhode Island	15	80
Wisconsin	Associated Hospital Service	149	34
Colorado	Colorado Hospital Service	8 (pilot)	36
Michigan	Michigan Hospital Service	12 (pilot)	58
Ohio: Cleveland area	Blue Cross of Northeast Ohio	2 (pilot)	56
Pennsylvania: Pittsburgh area	Blue Cross of Western Pennsylvania	17 (pilot)	56
Wilkes-Barre Area	Blue Cross of Northeastern Penn.	2 (pilot)	57

Table 3–2. continued *(Notes)*

Sources: Communication with Blue Cross Association, January 30, 1976; *Hospital Statistics*, 1975 ed. (1974 data from the American Hospital Association Annual Survey) (Chicago: American Hospital Association, 1975); Blue Cross Association Enrollment and Utilization Report, third quarter, 1975.

aBlue Cross plans in Delaware and New Mexico also have rate review and negotiating provisions in their contracts but are not included here because implementation, so far, has been minimal.

bVoluntary compliance.

Reprinted from Katharine G. Bauer, "Hospital Rate Setting—This Way to Salvation?" in Zubkoff, M., Raskin, I.E., and Hanft, R.S. (eds.) *Hospital Cost Containment: Selected Notes for Future Policy.* New York: PRODIST (published for the Milbank Memorial Fund in cooperation with the National Center for Health Services Research). 1978.

Table 3–3.   Hospital Rate Setting Activities of State Governments as of December 1975.

Name of State	Type of State Agency	Number of Hospitals Covered	Type of Payer Rates Currently Regulated	Estimated Share of Hospital Revenue Affected
Arizona[a]	Department of Health Services	75	Charges to self-pay patients Blue Cross	85
Colorado	Department of Social Services	89	Medicaid	8
Connecticut	Independent Commission	40	Charges to self-pay patients	30
Maryland	Independent Commission	54	Blue Cross Charges to self-pay patients	55
Massachusetts[b]	Independent Commission (full-time commissioners)	133	Medicaid; Charges to self-pay patients and others	45
New Jersey	Department of Health with concurrence Department of Insurance	104	Blue Cross Medicaid	55
New York	Department of Health with concurrence Department of Insurance; recommendation from Blue Cross plans	320	Medicaid Blue Cross	55
Rhode Island	State Budget Director with R.I. Blue Cross	15	Blue Cross Medicare Medicaid	90

| Washington | Independent Commission | 119 | Charges to self-pay patients Workmen's Compensation | 50–55 |

Sources: Telephone interviews with state agencies, December 1975; January 1976; *Hospital Statistics*, 1975 ed. (Chicago: American Hospital Association, 1975).

[a] Hospital rate review is mandatory under Arizona law, but compliance is voluntary. (To date there has been almost 100 percent compliance.)

[b] The Massachusetts Rate Setting Commission has approval power over the terms of Blue Cross contracts; since the current contract incorporates controls on charges consonant with the state's charge control law for self-pay patients, the 45 percent figure understates the commission's overall leverage.

Reprinted from Katharine G. Bauer, "Hospital Rate Setting—This Way to Salvation?" in Zubkoff, M., Raskin, I.E., and Hanft, R.S. (eds.) *Hospital Cost Containment: Selected Notes for Future Policy*. New York: PRODIST (published for the Milbank Memorial Fund in cooperation with the National Center for Health Services Research). 1978.

ment programs differ from the traditional retrospective cost reimbursement programs both because rates are set in advance and because an external body is involved in the rate determination process. The experience to date regarding the effectiveness of prospective reimbursement as a cost containment strategy must be interpreted cautiously. A major reason for this caution is that the evidence that exists is confounded by the effect of the Economic Stabilization Program, which became operational about the time that many of the early programs might have been having their initial impact. While, in most instances, evaluations of the prospective reimbursement programs do not show statistically significant savings, they are consistent with some small savings.[34]

There are many different rate-setting models, including complete review and negotiation of budgets; budget review by exception, which uses cost and productivity screens to identify components of hospital costs that appear to be particularly out of line; and formula-based methods that determine either allowable unit costs or allowable rates of cost increase and account for those environmental factors over which a hospital has no control.

Rate regulation may be difficult to implement effectively for hospitals because of the problem of measuring and comparing the products of different hospitals. Difficulty in measuring the product leads to difficulty in establishing the reimbursement rate. This administrative consideration is important in evaluating varying rate-setting processes. For states with a large number of hospitals, or for a national program, either a formula approach or a "budget review by exception" may be preferable to a negotiated budget approach. While the latter may be more sensitive to the variation in products and circumstances of individual hospitals, it is expensive and time consuming.

The formula approach to prospective rate reimbursement has been used in the state of New York since January 1970. New York's experience is particularly relevant to the administration's cost containment program, since each hospital in New York is allowed a growth rate in revenue reflecting price trends in the general economy.

New York uses formulas for Medicaid and Blue Cross plans that determine maximum allowable revenue per patient day. The per diem rate is allowed to grow at the same rate as an index of hospital input prices. Allowances for capital and charity costs per day are not permitted to rise over the base year, and allowable routine costs are derived from a classification system. Finally, the patient day base is subject to a lower limit of occupancy: 60 percent for maternity, 70 percent for pediatrics, and 80 percent for medical and surgical services.

After the introduction of the prospective reimbursement program in New York State, the rate of increase in hospital costs in that state went from a rate much in excess of the national average to a rate slightly below the national average. During this period, mean length of stay did not change appreciably either in New York State or in the country as a whole. This change in the rate of cost increase would thus appear to be attributable to the program itself and not to changes in the relative length of stay per admission. The growth in average cost per admission may also have been lessened, as suggested by the data developed by Berry and presented in Table 3–4.[35]

Table 3–4. Average Annual Percentage Increase, United States and New York State.

	United States		*New York State*	
Cost per admission				
1965–1970	14.1		16.5	
1970–1973	10.3		10.9	contains ESP period
1974	10.7		10.2	
Real inputs per admission				
1965–1970	7.6		9.2	
1970–1973	2.9		2.2	
1974	0.4		0.3	

The most interesting prospective rate-setting system from the standpoint of the current debate has been developed in Rhode Island.[36] In that state, the program objectives are (1) to contain costs, (2) to assure that growth in programs is based on statewide needs, (3) to shift resources away from inpatient care, (4) to reward efficiency and improve productivity, and (5) to ensure that cost control efforts do not have a deleterious effect on quality of care. The basic feature of the program includes a limit on total allowable operating expense increases on a statewide basis (MAXICAP). Within the context of this limit, each hospital budget is negotiated by Blue Cross, the State Budget Office, and the affected hospital. While the hospital guarantees the budget, provisions are made for ex post adjustments for volume increases and any major contingencies.

The program, which is voluntary, began in 1971; was suspended when ESP entered phase III; and was restarted in October 1974. During the first year, a MAXICAP of 13.85 percent was negotiated. Negotiated individual hospital budgets increased 12.58 percent in the aggregate. Actual increases were 15.2 percent, which were in excess of the negotiated rate and only a little below the national rate of 17 percent. The major causes of this disappointing experience were a disagreement about the purpose of volume corridors and a major unanticipated increase in malpractice insurance premiums.

For the second year (FY 1975–1976), the MAXICAP was 11.5 percent, while negotiated budgets were 10.5 to 11 percent. Although the actual increases are not yet known, the preliminary estimate of 12.6 percent is significantly below the national experience. For the 1976–1977 fiscal year, the parties negotiated a MAXICAP of 10.5 percent and an individual budget increase of approximately 10 percent.

The Rhode Island program has evolved within a cooperative atmosphere that has been aided by the small number of hospitals involved and the dominant position of Blue Cross. The major revisions that have been made in the program have included a redefinition of the major contingency provision, modification of the patient mix provision, and clarification of the use of gains derived from the volume corridor provisions. While extending the Rhode Island approach to a national program would most likely involve substantial implementation and administration difficulties, its approach does have some appeal as a cost containment measure.

Certificate of Need Legislation[37]

Previous efforts to control capital investment in the hospital industry have either been voluntary or (as in the case of Section 1122 of the 1972 amendments to the Social Security Act) have involved only minor sanctions for a capital investment undertaken without approval. Certificate of need (CON) legislation, however, is a major attempt to rationalize capital expenditures by hospitals. It remains to be seen whether the performance will live up to the promise.

Institutional health care providers have traditionally made their own resource allocation decisions. The only serious direct constraints on these decisions have been the availability of capital and the individual predisposition of those who participated in the decisions. The passage of CON legislation in certain states heralded the initial change in this relatively unrestrained freedom to make resource allocation decisions. The first CON acts were passed in New York in 1964, in Maryland and Rhode Island in 1968, and in Connecticut and California in 1969. They were alleged by their proponents to be responses to the rising costs of health care, to the purported oversupply of inpatient beds, and to an alleged unnecessary duplication of services. Although the strengths and weaknesses of such regulatory controls have been, and will continue to be, debated, there has emerged from these efforts experience in the United States with governmental regulation of capital expenditures by hospitals.[38]

The federal government became formally involved in the certificate of need concept with the passage of the Social Security Amendments of 1972. Section 1122 of that law permitted the states to designate state agencies to determine the appropriateness (in view of state plans) of a capital expenditure proposed by a health care organization. The strength of this approach lay in the fact that the Secretary of DHEW could control federal reimbursement for the costs attributable to the capital expenditure for the unneeded construction.

As of April 1974, thirty-seven states had conducted 1122 reviews; Blue Cross contracts in nineteen states included "conformance clauses," and direct CON controls had been legislated in twenty-four states.[39] The enactment in January 1975 of the National Health Planning and Resources Development Act of 1974 (PL 93—641) gave a strong new impetus to the certificate of need concept. Section 1523 of this act required that a state health planning and development agency, as one of its mandated functions, "administer a state certificate of need program which applies to new institutional health services proposed to be offered or developed within the state and which is satisfactory to the Secretary." This section of PL 93—641 also specified that the state health planning and development agency "shall consider recommendations made by a health systems agency."[40] In effect, the initial recommendation for the approval or disapproval of a new service must come from the local health systems agency, with a final decision being made at the state level by the state certificate of need agency. Clearly, the traditional freedom of health facility managers to make resource allocation decisions within their own organizations has now been limited. Both the administration and the Talmadge proposals would further shift the resource allocation decision away from the individual hospital to the health systems agency and to the state health planning and development agency.

Two major studies of CON performance have been completed, one by Hellinger, the other by Salkever and Bice. Hellinger, controlling for other determinants of investment, examined the effects on plant assets of both Section 1122 and CON laws using 1972 and 1973 state data.[41] He found that neither CON nor 1122 review exerted a significant influence on the level of plant assets. Hellinger also examined the data from the seven states that had passed CON legislation between January and September 1971 and a like group of seven that had passed legislation between January and September of 1972. His analysis indicated that hospitals in these fourteen states increased their levels of investment in anticipation of the laws' passage over the level of investment in states not passing CON legislation. One problem with drawing definitive conclusions from this type of analysis is the possibility of self-selection in the group of states passing CON laws. Furthermore, Hellinger's own analysis indicated that the rate of adjustment of plant assets was slow. It is thus not surprising that an examination of 1972 and 1973 plant assets finds that CON legislation passed in 1972 and 1973 has not significantly lowered hospital investment.

The more extensive investigation by Salkever and Bice examined the impact of CON on changes in total plant assets, assets per bed, and number of beds.[42] They chose the period 1968 to 1972 because Section 1122, the Economic Stabilization Program, and Blue Cross conformance clauses were less important in that time period than later. The hospital investment equation was estimated using data from non–CON states. Data from CON states were then applied to predict hospital investment, and the difference between actual and predicted investment was attributed to the effect of CON legislation.

Salkever and Bice found that CON had no significant effect on total hospital investment. Interestingly, CON was shown to reduce bed expansion, but to increase other plant investment. A similar examination of 1971–1973 data from a few selected Comprehensive Health Planning (CHP(B)) agencies showed no negative effect on bed supply and a positive impact on expansion of facilities and services. Finally, the effect of CON on hospital costs per patient day was investigated. Unit costs in CON states were found to increase, while days per capita and admissions per capita were reduced. The discovery that CON has actually acted to increase costs per patient day is a necessary corollary of the researchers' observation that assets per bed increased while bed expansion was restrained. Increased costs in this period may also be explained by the anticipatory behavior of hospitals; short-run increases in assets per bed are far easier to accomplish than the funding of major construction projects.

This picture of early CON performance is disappointing. A perspective on this early evidence can be gained by examining the functioning of CON programs in two states: Massachusetts and Maryland. The first nineteen months of Massachusetts' certificate of need program has been described by Bicknell and Walsh.[43] Formally instituted on June 1, 1972, the law applied to (1) all cases of original licensure, (2) capital expenditures in excess of $100,000, (3) the addition of four or more beds, and (4) substantial changes in service. The program is administered by the Public Health Council of the Commonwealth's Department of Public Health with participation by the applicant, the areawide CHP agency, and any group of ten or more taxpayers registered as participants and representing consumers, competing providers, and so forth. During the first nineteen months of operation, the council approved the addition of 5,247 beds, compared with 5,715 requested. Eighty percent of all facility improvement applications were approved. These data, however, do not include investments for which applications might have been filed had not providers anticipated rejection by the council.

Bicknell and Walsh provide us with a perceptive catalogue of the problems faced by CON agencies. These include:

1. Difficulty of establishing health system priorities. This is properly the job of a planning agency, not a regulatory body. The major flaw of many CON programs has been their lack of a formalized relationship with a state planning body. Massachusetts provided for the input of CHP(B) agencies but only in an advisory review and comment role. Thus, the Public Health Council had no standard to guide its decisions.
2. The taxing of agency resources. Ideally, the planning agency should be responsible for data collection, identification of health service needs, and establishment of health system priorities. Within this framework, the CON council should be able to weigh the subjective criteria submitted by the applicant and the need for innovation and flexibility. Lacking this substantial foundation, it is understandable that the Massachusetts Public Health Council found its resources to be strained. Although the law mandated a final decision within one year of application, 16 of 209 determinations were not completed as required. Such delays result in additional costs of construction. An outgrowth of this paucity of resources has been the tendency of CON agencies to focus on bed construction rather than expansion of services. Such a narrowed focus may explain the previously mentioned finding of Salkever and Bice that CON decreased bed investments but increased assets per bed. Indicators of adequate bed capacity are simply better developed than measures of program adequacy. This paucity of analytic and management resources is a problem that would need to be resolved before a program of hospital cost containment such as that proposed earlier in this volume could be successfully implemented.

3. Conflict of long-range system goals and short-term political implications. As Bicknell and Walsh state:

> State legislators who supported the bill when it was enacted have later
> tried to block its application to facilities in their districts. The genuine
> concern over rising costs of health care evaporates in the event of a threat
> to one's own community hospital.[44]

Rationalization of the health care system, to the extent feasible,
is a slow process and requires the coordination of regulation, planning and financing:

> Even with stringent standards, the long-range effects of determination of
> need will be felt slowly. The Public Health Council can examine the capac-
> ity only of hospitals petitioning for certificates of need, and the most rig-
> orous decisions yield but a minor bed reduction on paper in a given year.
> That reduction does not actually occur until the completion of approved
> projects some 3 or 4 years later. Furthermore, a denial does not remove
> existing beds from service, but merely prevents replacement or increase of
> existing capacity. Considerable lag time remains for adjustments.[45]

However, the fact that Salkever and Bice did find an effect on the
composition of investment implies that sufficient time had elapsed
for CON programs to have detectable effects. There is some evidence,
drawn mainly from the experience in New York State, that suggests
that a CON program that has been in existence for a longer period of
time may be associated with a small reduction in hospital investment,
at least enough to cover the administrative costs of the CON agency.[46]

Maryland's certificate of need program was established July 1,
1970, as an integral part of that state's Comprehensive Health Planning program (Steuhler, 1973).[47] CON is part of the requirement for
facilities to comply with the state's health plan. The program is administered by the state CHP agency with facility review delegated to
the areawide (B) agencies. Between July 1970 and April 30, 1972,
ninety-four decisions were made: three applications were disap-
proved, twelve approved with modification, and forty "small projects were not reviewed in detail."[48] Maryland's CHP staff was extremely overburdened, being responsible for licensure, planning, and
CON, and the state lacked the functioning network of areawide planning agencies envisioned by the CHP legislation.

Because so many CON programs have been conducted either under
the auspices of, or with input from, CHP agencies, it is important to
understand why this national health planning program has thus far

failed to have a significant impact. Three major sources of failure cited by O'Connor are:[49]

1. That the prerequisites for planning were not present at the time the legislation was passed nor could they be created by legislation. This generic deficiency in the whole planning process is underscored by Bicknell and Walsh when, in commenting on CON programs in Massachusetts, they state:

   Deficiencies manifest in certificate of need reflect a defect of government in general. Confronted by a long standing and worsening social problem— in this case how to put medical resources where they can serve people best —society takes virtually the sole recourse open to it and passes a law. But the passage of the law makes the problem no less complex. The implementation of the law calls on the same technology and social misunderstanding from which the problem originally issued.[50]

2. That neither the process nor the desired outcome of "planning for health" was specified. CHP agencies therefore lacked criteria by which to evaluate their progress.
3. That CHP agencies lacked the power to enforce their recommendations. Furthermore, their dependence on local providers for financing certainly led to a conflict of interest.

To these faults, Roseman added a tendency to avoid conflicts in policy formulation and a failure to deal with the root causes of health problems.[51]

The problems that the planning process in general, and now health systems agencies in particular, face in regard to allocation decisions are well illustrated in the current furor over computerized tomography (CT). CT, which has been called the first truly revolutionary recent innovation in radiology, is creating "technological shock" for the hospital industry.[52] The development of CT foreshadows the future development of other services about which allocation decisions will most likely involve HSAs. Computerized tomography "is a procedure whereby X-ray images of cross sections of the head or body (tomography) are reconstructed from numerous angles (axial) mathematically into three dimensions (by computer)."[53] The spread of this technology has been rapid. It was first introduced in 1972. There now exist nineteen different models (with six additional companies developing prototype equipment) with price tags ranging from $310,000 to $625,000. Beyond the initial capital outlay for the equipment, the cost of operation, including staff, is quite substantial.

Balancing this cost are a number of benefits:

1. Technical superiority over conventional diagnostic radiologic procedures. It discriminates between soft tissues having subtle density differences, and its high resolution capability permits an accuracy of diagnosis not previously available.
2. Reduced risk to patients. Radiation exposure may be less than that necessary with a conventional series of X-rays to achieve the same or better information. In addition, the procedure is non-invasive—that is, it is not necessary to insert catheters or dyes into a patient's vessels or organs. There is little discomfort, and the immediate, and often conclusive, results of the CT scan may often mean that the patient does not have to undergo more risky diagnostic evaluation—for example, craniotomy for head trauma. In one study at Toronto General Hospital, for instance, a review of 203 inpatients' and 241 outpatients' records showed that the information provided by a CT scan was sufficiently definitive that 170 pneumoencephalograms and 171 angiograms (which would have been necessary without the CT scan) could be avoided.[54]
3. Lower direct costs to some patients. In the Toronto General Hospital study, an estimated 328 inpatient days were saved. Using a per diem rate of $165, the authors calculated the savings at $264 per patient. When the savings resulting from doing CT scans rather than the conventional procedures were counted, the total savings rose to $60,088. Abrams and McNeil have presented preliminary data, however, which suggest that even though the use of the CT reduces the number of pneumoencephalograms and the like, its presence in an institution substantially increases the number of diagnostic radiology tests performed and hence can result in net increases in costs.[56]

For a technological innovation that has so many positive implications, the CT phenomenon has created a major dilemma in the health field—a dilemma that embodies many of the problems that will face health planners as they attempt to make decisions about new services in the health field. The dilemma is that of determining both how many CT units are needed in a given community and where they should be located. When the HSAs are fully operational, they will be expected to make such decisions on a rational basis. To date, the decisions made by existing planning agencies have often been inconsistent. For example, as Phillips and Lille point out with reference to CT scanners:

Jersey State Health Planning Council promulgated guidelines on January 1975 that recommended that certificates of need be granted for a total of six scanners, two for research and investigation at the medical schools and four for the rest of the state. This represents a ratio of 0.8 scanners per million persons. In contrast, the Comprehensive Health Planning Association of Imperial, Riverside and San Diego counties, in California, which has no certificate-of-need law, prepared a position paper in which they accepted a manufacturer's contention that the number of CAT scans done in a community should equal 1.5 times the number of brain scans. By this method, a maximum of seven units would suffice for the San Diego metropolitan area of approximately 1.3 million persons, a ratio of 5.4 cerebral scanning units per million persons.[57]

It is obvious that the basis upon which such an important resource allocation decision should be made has not been generally agreed upon. The current dilemma created by the CT technology will abate over time, but the basic problem of how the HSAs and certificate of need agencies should go about making similar decisions in the years ahead will remain. In summary, the performance record of the certificate of need program is limited and the impact mixed. Nevertheless, CON provides a critical mechanism for use within a cost containment program.

PSRO, Utilization Review, and Second Surgical Opinion Programs

The Professional Standard Review Organization (PSRO) provision in PL 92–603 attempts to assure effective, efficient, and economical delivery of medical care to Title V, XVII, and XIX patients. The law's aim is to reduce unnecessary medical procedures and to minimize length of hospital stay while encouraging physicians to use outpatient and extended care facilities. The CON program just discussed is related to the PSRO program insofar as CON provides a mechanism to adjust the supply of health facilities to correspond to the adjustment in demand that PSRO might produce.

The PSRO legislation is designed to permit the monitoring of the delivery of institutional care. This objective is accomplished through the establishment of a detailed review procedure. Each PSRO or hospital, if it is found to have an effective review process and is granted "delegated" status, is required to establish norms and criteria for hospital care. The norms are to be based on reasonable local patterns of practice and must be approved by a national standards review council. The norms and criteria developed are used by the PSRO coordinators in individual institutions to approve admissions, assign appropriate lengths of stay, and certify extensions of the initial length of stay, in an attempt to see that cases are handled in an efficient manner. The latter activities are collectively referred to as utilization review.

The results of research to date on the effectiveness of PSROs and utilization review in lowering rapidly rising costs have not been promising. A study by the Institute of Medicine concluded that there was no conclusive evidence that utilization review was cost-effective on average.[58] Although utilization review was found to be associated with decreased length of stay, the fixed costs associated with maintaining a bed were alleged to be of such a magnitude that it appeared doubtful whether the savings were sufficient to cover the costs of the review process. This study also questioned whether the medical care audit component of the PSRO legislation was associated with significant improvements in the quality of care. In addition, there appeared to be insufficient experience with the profile component of the legislation to render any verdict as to its efficacy. Interestingly, when the PSROs performed the utilization review themselves as compared to delegating the task to individual hospitals, the process was found to be less cost-effective. These higher costs could very well result from higher incremental overhead costs and from higher staffing ratios for the review process for PSROs as compared to hospitals.

Gertman examined termination of benefits as a result of utilization review in a case study of forty-four Massachusetts hospitals.[59] He found one termination per hospital per week. Many of these terminations were then transferred to nursing homes. He concluded that the process of review just about paid for itself and that, in the long run, it would not result in large cost savings.

Bluestone and Baugh and Brook and Williams examined utilization review in two other settings and concluded that the benefit-cost ratios were more favorable.[60,61] Bluestone and Baugh, however, made no allowances for the cost of alternate medical care and placements and used a high variable cost figure in their calculations.

An interesting, controversial, and potentially cost-effective form of utilization review has recently been developed in the provision of surgical care—namely, second surgical opinion programs. Spurred by concerns over unnecessary surgery as well as the rising costs of medical care, second opinion programs have spread dramatically over the United States in recent months. There now may be over fifty major programs. A number of these have been mandated by state legislatures for recipients of Medicaid and others have been set up by unions for their membership. In addition, the Department of Health,

Education, and Welfare has recently promulgated a national program to foster second opinions. Second opinion programs can be either voluntary or mandatory. In voluntary programs, a participant has the option of seeking a second opinion at no cost to himself when surgery is proposed. In mandatory programs, however, the consumer is required to obtain a second opinion (generally arranged by and paid for by the program), and this second opinion is generally a condition for receiving reimbursement for the proposed elective surgery. (Were a negative second opinion obtained, most programs would still reimburse the consumer if he decided to go ahead with the surgery.) Since there is substantial reason to believe that in voluntary programs a substantial preselection bias may exist and that a fair proportion of nonconfirmed cases might not have undergone surgery, even in the absence of a second opinion program, it would appear appropriate to focus on the results of evaluations of mandatory programs. McCarthy has accumulated the largest series of cases (1,145) from mandatory programs.[62] His latest results show a nonconfirmation rate among these 1,145 cases of 18 percent. Virtually the same proportion of cases are being reported as nonconfirmed in Massachusetts' recently mandated program for Medicaid recipients.[63]

A telephone followup by McCarthy of some of the nonconfirmed patients for periods of up to two years revealed that almost a third of those interviewed overrode the negative second opinion and went on to have surgery.[64] Almost half of these patients alleged a persistence or a worsening of their condition as the reason for their decision to have surgery. Were this proportion of override to be a generalizable property of the population of nonconfirmed patients, the net rate of deferred surgery in McCarthy's study would fall to 11 percent.

Given this apparent saving, it is important that the costs of such programs be rigorously analyzed to determine their net benefits. An accounting of the costs should include not only the direct costs of the second opinion but the time and travel costs of the patient, the cost of alternative medical therapy employed, and the psychic and social costs of the persistence of pathology in some proportion of the patients. Important benefits to be calculated include not only the direct costs deferred but the savings in pain, suffering, and iatrogenic complications obviated by virtue of the deferral of the surgery and any "sentinel" effect deriving from the existence of second opinion programs. McCarthy alleges such an effect in observing that the numbers of surgical claims being submitted for reimbursement to the steelworker unions decreased 9 percent from 1971–1972 to 1974–1975 as a result of their establishing a mandatory program. During this period, national surgical rates rose 20 percent.[65]

The Economic Stabilization Program

The Economic Stabilization Program (ESP) began in August 1971 with limitations on virtually all wages and prices. Both hospital prices and wage rates were controlled. The hospital sector continued to be covered by controls after they were lifted from most other parts of the economy (except energy) in 1973.

It is difficult to evaluate the effects of the price control part of ESP because any effects are necessarily confounded with the effects of wage controls. Since a hospital cost containment measure will typically not control wage rates (indeed, the administration's proposal permits a direct passthrough of costs associated with wage increases for nonsupervisory personnel), data from the ESP period can be used to evaluate the effects of revenue limits only by removing the consequences of wage controls from the data.

The pattern of changes in hospital costs and output before, during, and after ESP is indicated in Table 3–5. In the pre–ESP period, there was a large increase in hospital costs, primarily because of increases in inputs per adjusted patient day and per adjusted admission. The inflation rate began to drop after 1969, and declined at about the same rate during the ESP period. The rates of growth of labor input prices and in cost per adjusted admission were reduced somewhat during ESP. The reduction in the rate of increase in wage rates is likely attributable to the wage controls in effect during the ESP period, rather than to the price or revenue controls. Price controls could have served to stiffen a hospital administration's wage bargaining position or to reduce its willingness to grant "philanthropic" wage increases.

The most important determinant of the change in the inflation rate of costs per adjusted admission in this period was a decline in length of stay, but it is difficult to attribute the decline to price controls under ESP. Because hospitals were paid average rather than marginal costs under Phases II and III, and because the short-run marginal cost of additional days is usually well below average cost, there was no necessary incentive under ESP to reduce the length of stay. It is more likely that the changes in length of stay reflect other influences, such as utilization review. The data in Table 3–5 thus suggest that ESP itself had little effect on the rate of cost or expenditure increases. It did hold down the prices (e.g., the room rate) that hospitals charged, but greater use of other itemized services offset much of this effect.

The lack of a substantial effect of ESP on costs is confirmed by Ginsburg's econometric study of the ESP and pre-ESP periods.[66]

Table 3–5. Annual Rates of Increase, Selected Hospital Time Series.

	1963II^c–1966II	1966II–1969II	1969II–1971II	1971II–1973II	1973II–1975II	1975II–1976II	1976II–1977II
	Annual Rates of Change, Nominal Terms						
1. Expenses per Adjusted Patient Day	8.6	14.0	12.2	10.2	14.2	15.0	14.7[a]
2. Expenses per Adjusted Admission	8.4	16.7	10.0	8.2	13.9	14.8	10.0[a]
3. Revenue per Patient Day	8.9	14.1	12.6	9.3	16.5	16.0	15.9[a]
4. Revenue per Admission	8.7	16.7	10.2	7.3	16.7	18.7	11.2[a]
5. Full Time Equivalent Personnel per Patient Day	4.9	1.5	2.1	1.3	2.0	2.9	5.0[a]
6. Wage Rate per FTE personnel	—	9.5	7.2	6.6	8.9	8.1	7.4[a]
7. Hospital Cost Index (AHA)	—	—	7.5	4.1	10.6	10.0	7.5[b]
8. Hospital Intensity Index (AHA)	—	—	7.4	2.5	4.3	5.5	2.1
9. Consumer Price Index, Medical Care Only	2.9	6.7	6.4	3.6	10.7	9.5	9.8
10. CPI All Items Except Medical Care	1.9	3.9	5.0	4.8	10.0	5.5	6.5
	Annual Rates of Change, Real Terms						
1. Expenses per Adjusted Patient Day	6.6	9.7	6.9	5.2	3.8	9.0	7.7
2. Expenses per Adjusted Admission	6.4	12.3	4.8	3.2	3.5	8.8	3.3
3. Revenue per Patient Day	6.9	9.8	7.2	4.3	5.9	10.0	8.8
4. Revenue per Admission	6.7	12.3	5.0	2.4	6.1	12.5	4.4

[a]May 1976—May 1977.
[b]Not very reliable for 1977.
[c]II denotes 2nd quarter.

Sources: American Hospital Association Panel Survey (unpublished data); *Social Security Bulletin*, DHEW, April 1977.
Note: These figures differ from those in Table 3–1 because the data on which this table is based are from the panel survey sample rather than from the annual survey.

Using quarterly observations on census divisions for the period 1963–1973, Ginsburg concluded that there was no statistically significant effect on cost or revenue per patient day during the ESP period after adjusting for the effect of wage rates and other input price changes. There was a statistically significant but small effect on cost and revenue per admission, but even this effect disappeared when length of stay was added as an exogenous variable. Ginsburg speculated that the ESP had little effect for three reasons: (1) the ESP program offered no cost reduction incentives either for hospitals below the limit or for hospitals forced into a negative cash flow position; (2) the regulations were confusing and ambiguous; and (3) the controls were expected to be temporary.

Ginsburg's time series terminated in 1973. Following the cessation of ESP, there was a rapid increase in costs. If this period of rapid increase was prompted by the ESP controls, the evaluation of ESP turns critically on how one explains these increases. It could be argued that had it not been for the ESP controls, higher rates of increase would have occurred in the 1971–1974 period. From this viewpoint, the rapid increase in costs is the result of the eventual release of the cost-increasing pressures that ESP had repressed. Even if ESP were credited with keeping costs down, it is not obvious that the total (present value) of hospital cost inflation over the ESP and "bulge" or "catch up" periods was less because of ESP. What would have happened had the controls never been lifted is an important but moot point. One might also speculate that part of the "catch up," especially in the more recent period, might have been caused by anticipation of future price controls, an anticipation that was in part a response to the ESP experience itself. In this view, the ESP program may actually have made matters worse. It may have done more than just postpone inflation; it may have increased the total amount of inflation over the full period more than would have been the case without it.

The clearest conclusion of an analysis of the ESP period is that the temporary ESP controls did little good. The lessons learned from this experience are twofold: (1) controlling cost is not easy, and (2) if a cost containment program is to have a chance of success, it must be permanent and must be believed to be permanent.

The Canadian Experience

As national health insurance was introduced in all of the provinces of Canada, the initial policy was one of paying hospital costs, whatever they happened to be. Review took the form of a line by line examination of individual hospital budgets, resulting in a prospective budget from which adjustments were made at year end for substantial deviations between projected and actual costs. In general, such control as there was over hospital costs was exercised in the negotiations between provincial reimbursing agencies and individual hospitals. Wage increases were almost always passed through. On one occasion, however, the minister of health of British Columbia simply refused to approve the increases and, in Quebec, the government participates in wage negotiations.

As Evans notes, the primary deficiency in the budget review system was that, despite voluminous data inputs, budget reviewers had almost no information on outputs, not even on diagnostic mix.[67] The paying agency was willing to approve "appropriate" increases in budget, but no party knew how to define "appropriate." Evans suggests that budgeters fell back on incrementalism and rules of thumb. Between 1965 and 1971, hospital expense per patient day increased at an average rate of 15 percent, suggesting that this policy was not an effective constraint. Evans argues that the "inability of budget review to limit cost escalation has become more apparent."[68] Experiments in the form of fixed budgets, prospective budgeting, and incentive reimbursement have been tried, but without much success.

A more active policy gradually emerged in the 1970s in which the appropriateness of budgets was increasingly questioned. This policy was also not particularly successful in reducing the rate of inflation. While there was some slackening of the rate of inflation in the early 1970s, expense per patient day in Canadian public general hospitals increased by 19.8 percent and 17.9 percent in 1975 and 1976 respectively, rates even in excess of those in the United States for the same period.[69]

The current approach to controlling hospital expenditures in Canada appears to rely to a considerable extent on reducing hospital beds, in the hope that fewer beds will be associated with less use of hospitals. Canada has approximately 50 percent more beds per capita than in the United States and a higher admission rate. Such a policy will probably not reduce the rate of inflation in unit costs, but it may be successful in controlling total expenditures.

Chapter 4

Analysis of the Administration's "Hospital Cost Containment Act of 1977"

SUMMARY OF THE ADMINISTRATION'S PROPOSAL

The stated objective of the administration's proposal is "to curb the inflation in hospital costs, which is currently running far ahead of other prices, and to pave the way for more fundamental reform of the methods by which hospitals are paid and of the supply and distribution of health care services." The proposal alleges that two factors have led to this inflation: "The first factor is a third-party payment system that gives patients and their physicians little cause to consider hospital costs." The second is that "third-party payers reimburse hospitals on the basis of whatever the hospitals state as their costs, or whatever price the hospital charges."[1]

To deal with these market failures, the administration proposes "a transitional program . . . to bring the increase in hospital costs more in line with price trends in the rest of the economy." A transitional program is needed because "permanent structural reforms of the health care reimbursement system are expected to take up to three years to put in place." The program would apply to all "acute care and specialty hospitals" except chronic care institutions, new hospitals, HMO-funded hospitals, and federal hospitals.[2] The cost containment program contains two main features: (1) an "adjusted inpatient hospital revenue increase limit"[3] and (2) a national limit on capital expenditures by hospitals. "The cost-containment program would apply only to inpatient services because they represent the most expensive mode of treatment. The administration views as desirable shifts from in-patient to out-patient care when quality of care is maintained, since out-patient care is considerably less costly."[4]

The proposed formula for limiting inpatient hospital revenue reflects "general price trends in the economy as a whole, plus an additional amount to accommodate some increase in intensity of patient services." "The allowable increase would equal the increase in the GNP deflator for the most recently published 12-month period, plus 1/3 of the differences between the average annual increase in hospital costs in the preceding two years and the increase in the GNP deflator in that same period."[5] For a hospital that experiences an admissions level that is within +2 percent to −6 percent of its base year admissions, the revenue limit remains unadjusted. For changes in admissions levels outside this range, but not more than 15 percent, a hospital would receive 50 percent of the average revenue per admission for an increase in admissions, while for a decrease in admissions, revenue would be reduced by 50 percent of the average revenue per admission. Beyond the 15 percent range, no additional revenue would be permitted for admission increases unless an exception were granted, and full revenue reductions would be imposed for admission decreases except for small hospitals.

The program provides for exceptions to the revenue limit, the most important of which are (1) exceptional changes in patient load; (2) major increases in capacity or types of services, or major renovation or replacement of physical plant; (3) adjustment(s) based on actual increases in pay granted to non-supervisory employees; and (4) that hospitals which are located in states that have effective cost containment programs would be exempt from the federal program.

The base year for the application of this formula is 1976, so that hospitals would not be able to take any actions in anticipation of the program. Since the program has the potential of creating incentives that could lead to undesirable consequences, the program also contains a number of restrictions on hospital operations. For example, "hospitals would be required to maintain their charity patient load shares."[6]

The second principal component of the administration's cost containment program is a limit on capital expenditures by hospitals, to be enacted by amending the Public Health Service Act. The rationale for this component is that "a cost containment effort can only be effective over a long period of time if steps are taken now to slow the rate of growth of bed capacity and the duplication of expensive technology."[7] The permitted national limit on capital expenditures would be determined by the Secretary, but would not exceed $2.5 billion annually. It would apply to all capital expenditures, regardless of their financing. The limit would be allocated to states in the initial years on the basis of population, but in future years variations among the states in the costs of construction, population patterns and growth, and the need for hospital facilities and equipment could be taken into account. This supply ceiling would itself be limited by forbidding capital expenditures for beds in areas in which the ratio of four hospital beds per 1,000 population was exceeded or for which the occupancy rate was less than 80 percent. The capital expenditure limit is also coupled with a strengthening of the certificate of need legislation.

CRITIQUE OF THE ADMINISTRATION's PROPOSAL

Objectives and Perspectives

The purpose of this section is to analyze the specific provisions of the administration's proposal in order to illustrate the practical issues that underlie the design of any hospital cost regulation program. The aims of analysis are:

1. To assess whether the specific mechanisms in the proposal would promote the explicit objectives of the proposal, and
2. To assess the likely effects of specific provisions.

The explicit objectives of the proposal are to "curb the inflation in hospital costs," and to "pave the way for more fundamental reform."[8] In view of both the policy context of the administration's proposal and the likely permanence of some form of the legislation if it were passed, it would appear inappropriate to view the proposal solely in terms of its performance over the short run. It is more important that the proposed mechanisms be evaluated in terms of their long-run impact on the behavior of hospitals and on the performance of the health care delivery system.

The Revenue Limitation Formula

The formula for the maximum allowable increase in a hospital's inpatient revenue will first be analyzed under the assumption that the volume of admissions is constant from year to year. The formula proposed by the administration determines the percentages by which control year inpatient revenue per admission may exceed the base year inpatient hospital revenue per inpatient admission. The base year is 1976; the first control year is 1978.

The formula can be written in terms of the following symbols:

g_t = the maximum allowable increase in inpatient revenue in year t as a percentage of the base year.

p_{t-1} = the percentage increase in the implicit price deflator of GNP for year t-1.

r_{t-1} = the average annual percentage increase in total hospital expenditures during years t-1 and t-2.

π_{t-1} = the average annual increase in the GNP deflator during years t-1 and t-2.

The proposal specifies the formula as

$$g_t = p_{t-1} + 1/3\,(r_{t-1} - \pi_{t-1})$$

This formula limits a hospital's percentage revenue increase to a number beyond the control of an individual hospital. It neither rewards nor penalizes a particular hospital for having a lower (or higher) than average rate of increase in cost in the previous year. The formula is thus neutral with respect to hospitals that begin at different levels of expenditure in the base year; it does not deal with variations in the current level of expenditure nor does it attempt to treat efficient or inefficient hospitals differently.

Several aspects of this formula become more apparent if the GNP deflator is assumed to grow at a constant rate, p, for a number of years and if all hospitals are assumed to have revenue growth equal to the maximum allowable. In this case, $g_t = 2/3\,p + 1/3\,r_{t-1}$, where r_{t-1} is the annual average rate for the previous two years. (That is, $r_{t-1} = \sqrt{(1 + g_{t-1})(1 + g_{t-2})} - 1$ in view of the compounding for two years.) This relationship is depicted in Figure 4-1 by the solid line for the initial conditions of $g_0 = 15$ percent, $r_0 = 15$ percent, and $p_0 = 6$ percent, at time, $t = 1$.

The figure indicates that after five years, the growth of hospital revenues relative to the base would be virtually indistinguishable from the growth of the GNP deflator. However, because the formula utilizes the concept of a base year, the year to year rate of growth in revenues will be less than that illustrated by the solid line. The dashed line indicates the maximum allowable annual percentage increase in revenue per admission when the base year concept is used and when revenue per admission increases by 15 percent in both 1976 and 1977. (The proposal allows a transitional increase in 1977

Figure 4–1. Approach to Steady State Growth in Hospital Revenues.

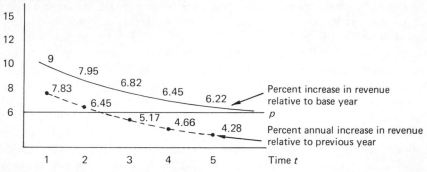

Percent increase in revenue per admission

over 1976 equal to the average rate of increase over the two years prior to 1976, but with a maximum of 15 percent and a minimum of 6 percent.)[9]

As illustrated, by the third year of the program, the allowable annual percentage increase is actually lower than the assumed increase in the GNP deflator. The conclusion to be drawn is that any cost containment program should address itself to the determination of the maximum allowable annual percentage increase in revenue. In the rest of our discussion, we shall define all references to revenue increase limits in terms of annual increases relative to the previous year.

With this assumption, the solid line can be used to illustrate the annual growth of hospital revenues. This annual rate of growth will eventually approximate the rate of growth of the GNP deflator. Such a situation is itself somewhat peculiar and is sharply different from the ordinary notion of "balanced growth," in which the revenue of one sector of the economy is a constant fraction of GNP. The rate of increase in the GNP deflator is equal to the difference between the rate of growth of money GNP (i.e., GNP in current prices) and the rate of growth of real GNP (i.e., GNP in constant dollars). Even if hospital revenues were permitted to grow at the rate of the GNP deflator, they would constitute not a constant but a declining fraction of money GNP, since real GNP grows at a long-run average rate of about 3 percent.

Under such a formula, the only increases in the intensity of services that would be permitted hospitals in the long run are those that could be realized by increased productivity in the provision of existing levels of services. A more reasonable approach, therefore, might be to permit increases in service intensity commensurate with the growth in real GNP. Specifically, if the GNP deflator is rising at 6 percent and real GNP is rising at 3 percent, increases in service intensity due to new facilities and programs could be permitted until revenue rises at a 9 percent rate. This would permit a constant share of hospital revenue in money GNP. (Such changes in capacity and intensity are explicitly provided for only through the exceptions stated in Section 115 of the administration's proposal.)

A further difficulty with the formula is that it does not relate, in the long run, to any policy parameters. The formula thus does not permit discretionary adjustments in the allowed rate of increase based on assessments of the appropriate level of expenditures for health, except by explicit legislative changes in the formula itself. It would appear that a cost containment program should permit policymakers more discretionary control of the key parameters of revenue limitations.

The "steady state growth path" in Figure 4−1 is of interest primarily as a target of the basic limit formula. It also serves to clarify the intended meaning of "curbing" hospital inflation. The choice of any truly exogenous target, as under the administration's proposal, would put a lid on real hospital inpatient revenue. A target of this type would be consistent with the view that hospital care has already become too large a drain on social resources and that the fraction of GNP devoted to it should be reduced. An alternative type of target that attempts to insure that the fraction of GNP going to hospitals is constant will be considered below presently.

In the case where the GNP deflator has a fluctuating growth rate, the basic limit in the administration's proposal requires hospitals to adjust gradually to a changing environment. To illustrate this property of the formula, a random variation in the GNP deflator (p_t) has been plotted in Figure 4−2, along with the resulting values of the maximum allowable percentage increase in revenue (g_t), if all hospital revenues grow at the maximum rate. The history depicted in Figure 4−2 indicates that, in a severely fluctuating economy, there would be years when hospital administrators would be severely restricted by the gradual adjustment formula. This potential problem has been anticipated to some extent in Section 112(b)(2) of the administration's proposal by allowing unexpectedly large increases in p_t to be inserted explicitly into the formula.

A principal difficulty in administering the formula is adjusting to the fluctuating prices of the inputs to hospital care, which are largely exogenous to an individual hospital. From year to year, the average price of inputs purchased by hospitals will change at rates different

Figure 4-2. Adjustment to a Fluctuating Target.

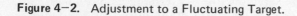

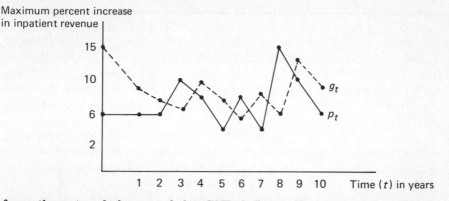

from the rate of change of the GNP deflator. For example, malpractice insurance premiums are believed to have increased at a rate of about 200 percent in 1975 alone. This increase probably had an exogenous effect on the unit cost of hospital services but undoubtedly had no observable effect on the GNP deflator.

Because of offsetting changes in the prices for individual items over a period of years, it may be expected that the cumulative change in the average price of hospital inputs would be close to changes in any general price index. However, during the interim years, hospitals would be required to adjust real purchases. While this sort of adjustment is technically feasible, it is likely to be inefficient. Therefore, serious attention should be given to the historical evidence on the year to year relationship between hospital input prices and the GNP deflator. This relationship is considered in the next subsection.

Hospital Input Prices and the GNP Deflator

In designing any formula for limiting hospital revenue, the basic objective should be to permit hospitals to obtain revenue to cover cost increases, such as increases in input prices, that are beyond their control and to force hospital decisionmakers and physicians who practice in hospitals to control those costs that are subject to their discretion.

Hospital inputs may be separated into nonlabor and labor categories. Each of these accounts for about half of hospital operating budgets. It is reasonable to assume that the prices of nonlabor inputs are exogenous to hospitals, but there is some question about whether wage rates are completely exogenous. Two decades ago, wages in the hospital industry were below those of comparable jobs elsewhere. They have risen substantially, however, and at present are higher than those for comparable nonhospital opportunities in many cases. The administration's proposal expresses concern that nonsupervisory employees not be made to "bear the brunt of the cost containment program." This concern is consistent with the view that hospital wage rates are not completely exogenous. Because the wages of nonsupervisory personnel have been specifically exempted from the revenue increase limit, we will consider only the prices of nonlabor inputs at this point. We will return in the next section to the subject of the labor cost exemption.

Two methods for calculating an index of nonlabor prices have been reported in the literature. Feldstein has developed an index for the years 1958–1967 based on inputs supplied by thirty-five different categories of industries.[10] The Bureau of Research Services of the American Hospital Association has more recently produced an index of nonlabor prices using weights from studies in New York and Massachusetts in the early 1970s.[11] Both the Feldstein and AHA indexes are reported in Table 4–1. The weighting factors from the AHA are reproduced in Appendix A.

Table 4–1. Comparison of Price Indexes.

Year	Hospital Nonlabor Price Index[a]	GNP Deflator	GPP Deflator
1958	1.000	1.000	1.000
1959	1.009	1.017	1.014
1960	1.023	1.033	1.028
1961	1.034	1.046	1.037
1962	1.044	1.058	1.047
1963	1.052	1.072	1.058
1964	1.064	1.089	1.071
1965	1.081	1.109	1.088
1966	1.109	1.139	1.116
1967	1.131	1.176	1.148
1967	1.000	1.000	1.000
1968	1.036	1.040	1.035
1969	1.081	1.090	1.083
1970	1.140	1.149	1.135
1971	1.188	1.202	1.182
1972	1.235	1.242	1.216
1973	1.338	1.312	1.286
1974	1.571	1.446	1.421
1975	1.897	1.693	1.677

[a]Sources: 1958–1967 from M. Feldstein, "Quality of Hospital Services: An Analysis of Geographic Variation and Intertemporal Change," in M. Perlman, ed. *The Economy of Health and Medical Care* (London: MacMillan, 1974); 1967–1975 from panel surveys compiled from American Hospital Association, unpublished data.

Over the sixteen-year period ending in 1973, there is a very high correlation between hospital nonlabor prices and the GNP deflator prices, even though, in the 1958–1967 period, the GNP deflator rises somewhat faster than input prices. A better year to year fit, however, appears to be obtained with the gross private product (GPP) deflator. One reason for this better fit might be that the GPP deflator does not include changes in government costs.

In 1974 and 1975, a major change took place in the relationship between the hospital input price index and both deflators. Both deflators began to underestimate the growth in the hospital index. The close historical relationship between the index and the deflators suggests that this divergence may be a temporary phenomenon. Nevertheless, the present size of the discrepancy is disturbing and implies that, under the administration's limit formula based on the GNP deflator, a significant amount of adjustment would have been required in the industry had the program been in effect in this period. Despite the apparent absence of an intention in the administration's proposal to maintain a constant real level of hospital inputs, it would seem advisable to cushion the industry against temporary and significant discrepancies between the GNP deflator and nonlabor input prices, such as malpractice insurance premiums.

On the other hand, a rationale for using a GNP deflator rather than an index that directly reflects nonlabor input prices paid by hospitals is that those prices may be administered by oligopolistic industries supplying hospitals. Hospitals have to date been reimbursed on a cost plus basis and thus, since consumers have had to pay only a small fraction of the true cost of care, hospitals have had little incentive to hold down the cost of inputs. As an example of the flexibility of certain input prices, it is widely believed that certificate of need legislation in Illinois reduced the price of a CT scanner below the $500,000 level simply because expenditures below that level were exempt from controls. The use of a broad deflator rather than a hospital industry deflator may encourage hospitals to exercise countervailing power against suppliers.

Labor Cost Exemption

Section 124 of the administration's proposal allows a hospital to obtain an adjustment in the maximum allowable growth of inpatient revenues if the wages of nonsupervisory personnel increase by more than the basic limit. This exemption is permitted until March 31, 1979, at which time it could be continued at the discretion of the Secretary.

Extensive analysis of reliable data has led several authors to conclude that hospital employees are no longer paid less than what they could receive in other industries. Indeed, by 1975 hospital wages in most job categories had "caught up" to, if not surpassed, wages of comparable positions in other industries. Using census data, Fuchs has shown that, by 1969, earnings of hospital employees were closely comparable to earnings of workers with equivalent sex, race, education level, and hours worked.[12] The Bureau of Labor Statistics also publishes wage data in which hospital and nonhospital wages may be compared in detailed job categories for metropolitan areas. A compilation of this data for 1960–1972 is presented in Table 4–2.

While the underlying motivation for the labor cost exemption in the administration's proposal may be political, there are two rationales for the exemption of nonsupervisory wage increases. The first is an objective that calls for a redistribution of income from relatively high income individuals to less highly paid individuals. It has been argued, however, that hospital nonsupervisory labor earns at least as much as in equivalent employment alternatives. The question then emerges whether the proposed exemption is an appropriate means for redistributing wealth and income or whether the general tax and transfer payment system might not be more effective. Most economists would agree that the latter system is a preferred means to accomplish wealth redistribution objectives.

The second rationale is that, without this exemption, nonsupervisory personnel would bear the brunt of the cost containment program. A number of studies have suggested that hospitals enjoy a monopsonistic position in local labor markets.[13] The alleged existence of such monopsony power was a common explanation for lower industry wage rates. (More recently, however, some have argued that hospitals have tended to take a philanthropic approach to employee compensation.[14]) It is impossible, however, to determine the extent to which hospitals can or will take cost reductions out of the wages of their low paid personnel. Given the growth of employee unionization, it seems unlikely that hospitals can be cavalier in their dealings with their work force.

For these reasons, the cost containment proposal presented in the earlier pages of this book does not include the exemption for nonsupervisory wage increases. It does, however, require the monitoring of the impact of the revenue limit on the low wage workers in the industry. Should it appear that the impact has been concentrated unfairly on this subgroup, the Secretary can make appropriate adjustments.

Table 4-2. Relative Wages of Hospital and Nonhospital Employees in Selected Occupations for Selected Metropolitan Areas, 1960–1972.

Metropolitan Area/Occupation	Hospital Wage as Percentage of Wage in All Industries				
	1960	1963	1966	1969	1972
Atlanta					
General duty nurse	73.6	73.2	81.9	94.7	93.8
Payroll clerk	—	—	92.2	103.3	104.4
Switchboard operator	72.5	67.9	80.0	89.7	91.5
Transcribing machine operator	95.3	—	—	108.4	107.0
Maintenance electrician	75.8	—	—	—	78.1
Stationary engineer	89.2	—	—	71.9	77.8
Porter	58.3	60.8	78.3	78.2	103.6
Maid	55.9	59.1	79.4	100.6	123.6
Baltimore					
General duty nurse	75.6	78.5	85.8	96.6	103.6
Payroll clerk	89.7	91.1	90.6	86.3	—
Switchboard operator	78.6	79.9	86.7	92.0	104.7
Switchboard-receptionist	67.7	66.4	—	103.6	100.5
Transcribing machine operator	85.6	91.8	107.4	111.3	119.7
Maintenance electrician	69.3	75.9	—	86.5	86.7
Stationary engineer	75.2	71.8	75.5	87.4	96.6
Porter	61.7	63.9	64.0	92.9	120.6
Maid	68.3	68.5	83.8	101.7	140.7
Boston					
General duty nurse	89.7	90.1	95.0	106.0	103.7
Payroll clerk	92.9	98.7	106.4	106.6	109.6
Switchboard operator	86.6	91.7	91.1	97.7	101.2
Switchboard-receptionist	—	85.9	—	—	102.2
Transcribing machine operator	96.2	98.6	96.8	99.5	109.1
Maintenance electrician	78.6	80.4	—	—	98.0
Stationary engineer	73.3	86.5	78.9	80.2	88.4
Porter	72.5	75.6	86.5	96.5	102.5
Maid	82.5	89.0	89.9	107.2	112.9
Chicago					
General duty nurse	91.4	91.3	95.2	105.0	103.3
Payroll clerk	84.8	89.7	99.5	88.7	103.3
Switchboard operator	79.5	82.5	90.3	96.2	101.3
Switchboard-receptionist	—	75.9	—	—	103.3
Transcribing machine operator	96.2	95.6	102.9	109.5	116.4
Maintenance electrician	86.6	87.0	—	—	100.0
Stationary engineer	88.6	87.8	90.7	90.1	88.8
Porter	64.4	68.6	72.1	85.5	96.5
Maid	67.5	71.4	76.0	89.6	103.0
Dallas					
General duty nurse	84.6	86.5	88.1	97.1	105.1
Payroll clerk	89.4	91.7	88.6	85.6	97.9
Switchboard operator	79.4	77.2	86.3	86.1	87.6
Switchboard-receptionist	—	—	—	—	84.0
Transcribing machine operator	100.8	103.9	102.0	106.1	111.1
Maintenance electrician	70.0	—	—	—	96.2
Stationary engineer	75.6	95.1	96.4	92.6	93.5
Porter	70.5	75.7	83.4	89.4	103.9
Maid	72.1	87.6	89.4	94.1	120.1

(Table 4-2. continued overleaf)

Table 4–2. continued

Metropolitan Area/Occupation	Hospital Wage as Percentage of Wage in All Industries				
	1960	1963	1966	1969	1972
Los Angeles					
General duty nurse	83.3	83.7	87.3	101.0	108.0
Payroll clerk	83.7	90.2	88.9	97.1	96.6
Switchboard operator	83.7	85.5	90.4	102.3	98.2
Switchboard-receptionist	84.7	82.7	—	—	97.5
Transcribing machine operator	108.7	109.4	107.2	118.5	113.6
Maintenance electrician	93.1	85.5	—	—	87.9
Stationary engineer	79.2	75.9	84.4	92.3	89.4
Porter	73.7	77.8	79.02	85.4	89.9
Maid	76.5	78.9	76.4	82.4	93.9
New York					
General duty nurse	83.9	88.1	99.2	111.1	116.1
Payroll clerk	85.6	93.3	102.5	102.6	108.7
Switchboard operator	84.1	87.1	93.8	100.5	113.7
Switchboard-receptionist	76.6	—	—	91.3	108.3
Transcribing machine operator	97.2	104.4	106.2	112.9	119.1
Maintenance electrician	79.4	84.4	—	90.6	100.2
Stationary engineer	84.5	95.8	99.7	113.1	109.0
Porter	67.2	78.8	81.0	91.7	105.4
Maid	75.0	88.4	91.4	102.5	110.2
St. Louis					
General duty nurse	—	—	84.1	132.5	97.7
Payroll clerk	—	—	86.2	94.3	92.5
Switchboard operator	—	—	81.2	92.2	100.3
Switchboard-receptionist	—	—	—	—	—
Transcribing machine operator	—	—	86.1	91.0	103.6
Maintenance electrician	—	—	—	—	82.2
Stationary engineer	—	—	70.9	80.2	90.4
Porter	—	—	66.4	77.6	77.1
Maid	—	—	90.7	96.7	97.8
San Francisco					
General duty nurse	86.5	86.0	77.9	104.4	76.6
Payroll clerk	101.1	87.0	100.9	90.0	103.7
Switchboard operator	95.3	101.8	105.1	100.9	117.5
Switchboard-receptionist	95.2	91.0	—	92.3	—
Transcribing machine operator	104.0	112.7	116.9	107.3	126.6
Maintenance electrician	—	—	—	93.5	—
Stationary engineer	88.7	91.3	95.8	91.1	105.6
Porter	75.8	78.0	82.5	85.9	100.0
Maid	78.8	79.4	83.2	86.3	98.8

Source: M. Feldstein and A. Taylor, "The Rapid Rise of Hospital Costs," Harvard Institute of Economic Research, Discussion Paper No. 531, 1977.

Note: — indicates that data are not available.

The Admissions Load Adjustment

The other major adjustment to the inpatient revenue increase limit in the administration's proposal is a method of responding to changes in the level of admissions. For any hospital, if the number of admissions is within +2 percent and −6 percent of the base year, the permitted increase in total inpatient revenue is equal to the allowable limit (e.g., 9 percent) applied to the base year revenue. For smaller hospitals, admissions may fall by 10 percent without reducing revenue. If admissions increase by more than 2 percent, hospitals will receive 50 percent of base period revenue per admission for each extra admission. If admissions decrease by more than 6 percent, revenue is reduced by 50 percent of base period revenue per admission for each admission below 6 percent. These adjustments are limited to a ± 15 percent change in admissions interval.

The analysis of these rules is aided by Figure 4−3. In this figure, it is assumed that the basic limit on revenue increase is 9 percent in the particular year, and the maximum allowable revenue is plotted as a function of the number of admissions. The exact formula, letting R stand for revenues, A for admissions, and the subscripts $0, 1$ for the base year and current year, respectively, is:

$$R_1 = R_0 + 0.5 \; \frac{R_0}{A_0} \; (0.13 A_0), \text{if } A_1 > 1.15 \, A_0$$

$$R_1 = R_0 + 0.5 \; \frac{R_0}{A_0} \; (A_1 - 1.02 A_0), \text{if } 1.15 A_0 > A_1 > 1.02 A_0$$

$$R_1 = R_0, \text{ if } 1.02 A_0 > A_1 > 0.94 A_0$$

$$R_1 = R_0 - 0.5 \; \frac{R_0}{A_0} \; (0.94 A_0 - A_1), \text{if } 0.94 A_0 > A_1 > 0.85 A_0$$

$$R_1 = R_0 - 0.5 \; \frac{R_0}{A_0} \; (0.09 A_0) - \frac{R_0}{A_0} \; (0.85 A_0 - A_1), \text{ if } 0.85 A_0 > A_1$$

For example, if admissions rise by 5 percent, revenue would rise by 10.575 percent rather than 9 percent. If admissions fall by 10 percent, revenue would rise by only 7.865 percent. While the parameters of this formula are inherently arbitrary, it is clear that hospital revenue should not be independent of the number of admissions, since short-run costs will be a function of admissions.

Unfortunately, the evidence on the relationship between the short-run incremental costs and average costs is inconclusive. In an early

Figure 4–3.   Maximum Hospital Inpatient Revenue in Current Year.[a]

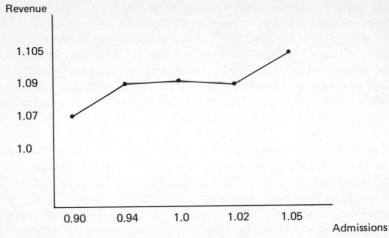

[a]Revenue and admissions in prior year have been normalized to 1.

study P. Feldstein, using monthly data, estimated that short-run marginal cost is only 20 percent of average cost.[15] Most other hospital cost studies have estimated long-run rather than short-run marginal cost and have found that long-run marginal cost is a much larger percentage of average cost.[16] In fact, a recent study of hospital costs using the more flexible translog formulation of the joint cost function estimated marginal cost of each output to be substantially greater than average variable cost.[17] If the true short-run marginal cost is below the amounts implied by the parameters in the administration's proposal, hospitals will experience either financial distress or windfalls of net revenues.

While the administration's proposal is temporary and is directed to controlling short-run costs, volume changes ultimately have long-run effects. Long-run decreases in volume should lead to structural changes in the provision of care in a hospital. These changes would involve decreases in available beds, reductions in services that can more economically be provided at other hospitals, and reductions in personnel at both the supervisory and nonsupervisory levels. Long-run incremental costs are closer to average costs than are short-run incremental costs and certainly are higher than the 50 percent figure specified for changes outside the −6 to +2 percent corridor. As a result, application of the short-run admissions adjustment formula will not be consistent with the long-run cost structure of hospitals. Hospitals with increasing admissions may not be able to generate sufficient revenue to cover the cost of providing the greater level of care with the 50 percent limit, while hospitals with decreasing admissions may be able to reduce costs by more than the 50 percent reduction imposed on them. The short- and long-run effects of the formula are thus potentially quite different.

It is therefore desirable to institute a long-term policy rather than a series of short-run policies. Short-term policies may function effectively for a while, but they would create, in the long run, an excessive burden on hospitals in growing areas and would provide windfalls to hospitals that are experiencing decreases in output. The administrations's interim proposal is likely to fail if it is applied in successive years. If such a program is to become permanent, the formula should be adjusted to better match the long-run cost structure of hospitals. Methods will need to be devised to distinguish between output changes that are expected to be temporary and those that are expected to be permanent.

Admission and case mix changes cannot be forecast with precision, and hospital management should not be expected to be able to alter dramatically the level of admissions, which is largely determined by physicians and the health of their patients. Therefore, a range of variation should be tolerated before invoking adjustments in the revenue limit. The need for adjustments in circumstances of an increasingly costly case mix are recognized in Sections 102 (d) and 115 (a) (2) of the administration's proposal. This adjustment is, of course, an asymmetrical approach to the sharing of risks, but at least it protects a community somewhat from untoward alterations in its hospitals' budget.

The Revenue Limit and Third Party Payers

Compliance with the volume load formula increases the already substantial administrative load required by the basic revenue limit. During a given year, a hospital will be collecting revenue from several sources. The administration's proposal requires the collection of this revenue during the year as if total admissions were to be unchanged. More specifically, if revenue per admission from one source, (e.g., Medicare, Medicaid, "cost payers," or "charge payers") in the previous year is given by R and the growth limit is g, this payer may be billed up to $(1+g) R$ in the current year. At the end of the current year, admissions will most likely not be equal to the base year total. There would typically be a need to credit or debit accounts for the next year with each payer or to arrange a cash settlement. Such settlements are now a common practice for cost payers. For non-cost payers, the administration's proposal provides for an escrow account in order to facilitate year to year reconciliation. This procedure deals with the problem equitably for classes of payers, although it does not compensate individual patients, especially those who pay out of pocket.

The services of physicians are an integral part of the care that a hospital inpatient receives. Two major categories of physicians may be identified by type of services produced: physicians directing the treatment of a specific patient and physicians producing laboratory, radiologic, or other supporting services. These two categories will be called attending and supporting physicians.

Attending physicians are not ordinarily paid by a hospital. Although attending physicians bill patients and third parties directly, they have a definite financial stake in hospital resources and procedures. Hospital resources influence the productivity of an attending physician's time by influencing both the qualitative nature of his output per unit of time and the time requirement per case. Specialized nonphysician personnel in hospitals reduce physician time per case, and capital investment in diagnostic and treatment facilities tends to increase physician productivity. Accordingly, one should not overlook the pecuniary interest of attending physicians in both the availability of and the pricing of hospital services. An effective lid on the expansion of service intensity in a hospital may cause greater investment by physicians in office-based care, ceteris paribus. This particular development may also result in smaller total cost increases than otherwise would have occurred. In office-based practice, there is likely to be greater cost consciousness by the individual physician. Such a shift, however, could also result in the exemption of the use of critical resources from controls.

One should perhaps be more concerned, however, about the effect of cost containment proposals on the relationship between hospitals and supporting physicians. Pathologists, radiologists, and anesthesiologists may be paid within or outside a hospital budget. For example, in 1969, only about 27 percent of hospital-based pathologists and a similar fraction of radiologists billed patients independently. A large volume of the services of these physicians could be divorced from hospital budgets. For a cost containment program to be effective, there must be a provision for systematically adjusting a hospital's revenue limit in response to such a shift.

The administration's proposal does contain such a provision for adjusting revenue downward if salaried physicians are replaced by a fee for service arrangement. The proposal does not appear to permit an increase in the base if physician compensation is changed from fee for service to inclusion in the hospital's charges. Our recommended cost containment program does contain the latter provision.

The Exemption of Outpatient Care

The administration's proposal exempts hospital outpatient revenues from control. To predict the effects of this exemption, it is necessary to examine the role of outpatient care in the medical care system. Outpatient departments of hospitals serve two roles. In part they are complementary to the hospital's inpatient care, since procedures related to an inpatient hospital episode but done either before or after the episode can be performed in outpatient departments. In part, however, outpatient departments are substitutes both for inpatient care and for physician office practices. The extremely rapid growth of hospital outpatient visits is primarily the result of substitution of hospital services for private practice physician services, either when there is no regular physician or when the regular physician is not available. Particularly for families in low income neighborhoods, the hospital outpatient department is the source of primary care.

Hospital outpatient departments are usually said to operate at a loss, when revenues are compared to fully allocated costs. However, it is not known if revenues cover marginal cost or whether additional outpatient visits increase revenues elsewhere in the hospital. If outpatient departments do generate losses at the margin, then it is very unlikely that hospitals will wish the quantity of such visits to expand if inpatient revenues are limited. Holding revenue per visit constant, an increase in the number of outpatient visits will impose even greater losses on the hospital. Indeed, if the limitations on inpatient revenues reduce hospital net income from some "profitable" inpatient departments, it is likely that hospitals will want to reduce their outpatient services, since deficit operations will have to be cut in response to controls.

If, on the other hand, hospital outpatient departments yield revenues equal to or in excess of the costs attributable to them, then they may serve as an outlet for the output maximization revenue or service intensity desires of administrators frustrated by inpatient revenue controls. To some extent, the commitment of resources to outpatient settings may be desirable, since switching patients from inpatient to outpatient care may lower costs, and the provision of additional primary care to populations in which there is excess demand may be worthwhile. The danger is that outpatient department expansion may not provide new "needed" care. Instead, such departments may provide unneeded care in too expensive a manner or, in certain situations, may further displace private office practices. Since the latter are generally less expensive, such a shift, to the extent it occurred, may actually increase total costs.

It is also possible that hospitals interested in maintaining total revenue and total output will switch some procedures to outpatient departments and load as much of their increased costs as possible on the unregulated outpatient departments. For example, if a hospital wishes to add a new service, but is prohibited from doing so by the inpatient revenue limits, it may still be able to add the service if it can have some or all of the service used by persons classified as outpatients—for example, either before or after the inpatient stay. This has both desirable and undesirable aspects. The desirable aspect is that, if the service is to be used, it may be less expensive not to hospitalize the patient who uses it. An undesirable aspect is that the service may be excessive in the first place. The comparative cost disadvantage of inpatient care versus outpatient care may be exaggerated, however, since the shift of a patient from an inpatient to an outpatient setting can cause substantial indirect and unreported costs. A sick person must be cared for, housed, and fed even if he is treated as an outpatient, and such treatment may also require others to spend time taking him to the hospital.

The effect of the exemption of outpatient care on the price and costs of that care is even less clear, since the outpatient pricing behavior of hospitals varies considerably. It is possible that outpatient charges are not higher because the outpatient department would then price itself out of the ambulatory care market, especially since out of pocket payments meet a more significant portion of the cost of outpatient care. Reduction in the availability of inpatient care may increase outpatient demands and push up prices. Costs may also rise as well, particularly if physician time for outpatient departments is in short supply and must be more heavily rewarded.

In summary, it is likely that the exemption of outpatient care will increase the demand for outpatient care and consequently the price of such care. Substitution of outpatient for inpatient care seems generally desirable and will be encouraged by the exemption. If hospitals turn to their outpatient departments to satisfy their desire for revenue and service expansion, however, the outcome may not be so desirable. There will at least be a temptation to use the flexibility of accounting procedures to shift revenues from inpatient to outpatient accounts. It is for these reasons that we have not exempted outpatient care from our cost containment program.

The Solvency Exemption

In an attempt to relieve individual hospitals from a threat to their existence, the administration's proposal gives the Secretary authority to grant exceptions from the limits. In order to qualify for an exception, a hospital must prove either (1) that its costs have exceeded the base year costs as a result of an admission increase of more than 15 percent or (2) that changes in the capacity of, or in the character of, the services rendered by the hospital or major renovation or replacement of physical plant have resulted in cost increases more than one-third of the difference between the average annual rate of increase in total hospital expenditures for the previous two years and the annual rate of increase in the GNP deflator in the previous two years; and (3) that the hospital is in danger of insolvency because its current ratio of assets to liabilities is below the 25th percentile of all hospitals, and (4) that the changes in admissions, capacity, plant, or services have had, and will continue to have, a certificate of need approval.[18]

If the hospital proves the above and the Secretary grants an exception, the hospital must make itself available for an operational review by the Secretary. The findings of the review will be made public, and the continuance of the exception shall be contingent on implementation of plans for improvements in the hospital's efficiency and economy.

If the hospital obtains an exemption because its admissions changed beyond the 15 percent limit, it can continue to receive 50 percent of the basic revenue for each additional admission beyond the limit. If it receives an exemption because of changes in capacity, character of services, or modernization, it is permitted to increase its revenue by an amount sufficient to bring its current ratio up to the 25th percentile and to maintain the ratio at that level.

One of the critical issues to be addressed in designing a regulatory program is how extensive the exceptions process should be. An extensive exceptions process, under which a large number of those regulated will qualify, will require a substantial administrative capacity to deal with applications in an equitable and expeditious manner. A less extensive exceptions process, while easier to administer, runs the risk of inflicting harm in certain atypical institutions.

The administration's proposal applies across the board revenue limits that are not sensitive to an individual hospital's circumstances. The requirements of the exceptions process are severe and, it might be argued, amount to a de facto "no exception" process. It does not seem unreasonable to expect that some hospitals that are in real financial difficulty (for example, with a current ratio well below the 25th percentile) would not qualify for an exception because they have neither an admission change beyond 15 percent nor changes in capacity, character of services, renovation, or replacement.

On the other hand, those hospitals that partly qualify under the exceptions process have an incentive to manipulate the rule to their benefit. In effect, this process may create incentives for some hospitals that satisfy the other criteria to become "insolvent" in order to subsequently acquire added revenue. This behavior, as well as the exceptions process itself, could have profound effects upon the market for hospital debt. At a minimum, it would increase the risk to the lenders and consequently the interest rate demanded. One way of avoiding these problems is to introduce within the cost containment proposal a mechanism for allocating both capital expenditures and operating costs that is more sensitive to individual hospital circumstances. The program we have outlined contains such a mechanism.

There is another problem with the solvency exemption in the administration's proposal. Given the wording of the proposal and, of course, the interpretation that the Secretary gives to this wording in the regulations for implementation, it is possible that a hospital could find itself in the following paradoxical situation: it could be practically insolvent, while not technically insolvent—that is, not qualifying for exception consideration under the solvency provision of the bill. This problem arises from the definition of working capital (see Section 115). No distinction is made between cash and marketable securities that are restricted in principal and/or income for purposes other than operating cost. Consequently, a hospital with large restricted endowments may be above the qualifying solvency ratio set by the Secretary, but not have sufficient funds to actually pay its debts (i.e., insolvent). Changing the bill to read all unrestricted cash, marketable securities, and so forth, would avoid this possible technical problem.

Finally, it should be noted that the measure of solvency contained within the administration's proposal (i.e., a current ratio below the 25th percentile) is arbitrary. The problem would be less critical if "solvency" were easier to measure. Unfortunately, reality is more complex and argues again for flexibility in the interpretation of the circumstances of individual hospitals.

Analysis of Title II—Limitation on Hospital Capital Expenditures

To avoid duplication of services and to limit the expenditure for new technology, the administration's proposal contains a program designed to limit hospital capital expenditures by imposing a national limit on such expenditures.

The National limit would be allocated to the States by a formula based on population for at least the first year. In later years, the Secretary could adjust the formula to take into account factors other than population—such as costs of construction and need for capital expansion or moderni-zation. . . . Second, in any health service area in which the number of hos-pital beds exceeds 4 per 1,000 population, or in which the average hospital occupancy rate is less than 80 percent, no certificates of need would be allowed if they would yield a net increase in beds in the area.[19]

As indicated in Chapter 3, certificate of need legislation has had some effect on limiting the growth in beds, but it has had little effect on the rate at which hospitals acquire new technology. Restrictions on bed supply may well be warranted, and the capital expenditure limit should be effective in limiting such future growth. The most desirable reduction in capital expenditures, however, may be in those used for the acquisition of new medical technology.

Placing a dollar limit on capital expenditures might not only con-trol the rate of expansion in technology, services, and facilities, but also make the opportunity cost of approval of a project more obvi-ous. Planning with a budget constraint should be a more rational and meaningful process than planning without the explicit consideration of foregone opportunities.

While a national limit on capital expenditures may well be appro-priate, there are two primary problems associated with the limit. First, the $2.5 billion upper limit proposed for the first year is arbi-trary. The present state of knowledge does not permit an explicit determination of a "best" limit. The legislation would be improved, however, if it could include a mechanism that would allow for the level to be adapted to the level at which marginal benefits may ap-proximately equal marginal costs. Such a mechanism might involve HSAs and other local certificate of need organizations. They are not staffed, however, to play such an increased role. The difficulties in-volved with the administration of certificate of need programs were illustrated in Chapter 3, and the need for additional resources to en-able HSAs to function more effectively in the area of cost contain-ment was addressed in Part I of this volume.

The second problem in administering the capital expenditure limi-tation lies in the exclusionary provisions. These provisions are based on the current bed supply in a community and on the current occu-pancy rate. This restriction comes very close to preventing any new investment in beds. Based upon information in the 1975 *Hospital Guide Issue*, these restrictions would prevent investment in new beds in all but two of the one hundred largest cities (fifty-eight of which have an occupancy rate below 80 percent, and all but two of those with occupancy rates over 80 percent have greater than four beds per

1,000 population). Similarly 244 of 297 SMSAs would be unable to invest in beds. In forty-eight of fifty states plus the District of Columbia, the occupancy rate for nonmetropolitan areas is below 80 percent. (The exceptions are New York and New Jersey.) These restrictions would appear to be too stringent, and an element of flexibility as contained in our cost containment program would appear appropriate.

When there is a "genuine" excess of hospital beds in a given area, it may be appropriate to do more than prevent the construction of additional beds. Accordingly, the certificate of need agency should also be authorized to carry out, at its own initiative, a program of bed decertification. Our cost containment program contains provisions establishing a mechanism both for decertification and for meeting the costs of such decertification.

A potential deficiency in Title II is the exclusion from the certification of need process of capital expenditures made outside the hospital setting. This is a particularly severe problem with regard to the acquisition of equipment by physicians in private practice for their offices or, in some cases, for space rented from the hospital. If it makes sense to control the rate of increase in the intensity of care, then it would appear appropriate that such controls apply to the entire health system. The implementation and monitoring of such a program, however, would appear to represent a complex problem for which procedures or standards do not exist. Accordingly, we have not at this time included such a recommendation in our hospital cost containment program.

Chapter 5

Summary and Analysis of
the Talmadge Proposal

INTRODUCTION

The legislation introduced by Senator Talmadge contains four major sections: (1) hospital reimbursement, (2) practitioner reimbursement, (3) long-term care, and (4) revisions in the administrative structure of the Medicare and Medicaid programs. In this analysis, we will concentrate on hospital reimbursement.

The major features of the legislation dealing with hospital reimbursement are (1) a mechanism for incentive reimbursement by Medicare and Medicaid for hospital "routine operating costs" and (2) a set of proposals that specify a hospital's eligibility for cost and/or incentive reimbursement.[1] The latter changes would restrict transfers of costs in excess of Medicare and Medicaid allowable costs to other third party payers, tighten the criteria for nonallowable costs, and provide procedures for dealing with metropolitan areas that cross state boundaries. The major innovative feature of the hospital reimbursement sections deals with incentive reimbursement for routine operating costs. This chapter will focus on this last aspect of the bill.

The underlying rationale of the incentive reimbursement provision is the desire to reward those hospitals that are efficient by permitting them to share in savings they generate when their routine operating costs are at a level below a prospectively set amount. To administer this program, hospitals are to be classified according to bed size, by type of hospital, and by "other criteria which the Secretary may find appropriate, including modification of bed-size categories."[2] The system will not, however, distinguish between hospitals on the basis of ownership. The three types of hospitals to be differentiated are "short-term general hospitals," "hospitals which are the primary affiliates of accredited medical schools" (these hospitals would not be classified according to bed size), and "psychiatric, geriatric, maternity, pediatric, or other specialty hospitals."[3] For each class of hospital, a per diem payment rate would be established equal to "the average per-diem routine operating cost amount for the category in which the hospital is expected to be classified during the subsequent fiscal year."[4] This per diem payment rate would be used to determine payments only for those patients covered by Medicare and Medicaid. To facilitate measurement of the appropriate costs on a comparable basis across hospitals, the bill proposes the establishment of "an accounting and uniform functional cost reporting system (including uniform procedures for allocation of costs)."[5]

THE INCENTIVE REIMBURSEMENT SYSTEM

The incentive reimbursement mechanisms would be desirable if the cause of the high level of hospital costs were the inefficiency of individual hospitals. Such an inefficiency would presumably take the form of excess beds, excessive staffing, poor coordination within the hospital, and other forms of waste and duplication. As indicated earlier, such technical inefficiency may contribute to an explanation of the high level of hospital costs, but it cannot explain the high rate of increase in costs unless hospitals as a group are becoming increasingly more inefficient over time. This latter possibility cannot be ruled out completely, because hospitals have been expanding their services and the range of their medical technology, but a more plausible hypothesis, as advanced previously, is that the insurance system has reduced the cost to consumers to such a level that they demand an excessive amount of medical care and an excessive level of services. On the supply side, hospitals have a desire to expand their services and to obtain the latest technology. An additional cause both of the high level of hospital costs and of the rapid rate of increase in costs is that the catch up wage policy of the 1960s has continued, so that hospital employees now are paid more than comparably skilled employees in the private sector. If these are the underlying causes of the problem, causes that do not involve technical inefficiency and that are primarily concerned with ancillary rather than routine costs, it is difficult to see how the Talmadge bill will alleviate the problem of inflation. In summary, the Talmadge bill provides incentives for greater hospital efficiency, but individual hospital inefficiency does not appear to be a major cause of inflation.

The costs to be covered by the incentive reimbursement system are those designated as "routine operating costs." These are defined to exclude the following: "(A) capital and related costs, (B) direct personnel and supply costs of hospital education and training programs, (C) costs of interns, residents, and non-administrative physicians, (D) energy costs associated with heating and cooling the hospital plant, (E) malpractice insurance expense, or (F) ancillary service costs."[6]

A per diem payment rate for routine operating costs would be determined by (1) grouping hospitals according to the classification system, (2) calculating the average per diem routine operating cost within each group of hospitals, and (3) determining the per diem payment rate for each hospital in the group by adjusting the personnel cost component of the average cost per day to reflect the difference in wages in the specific hospital's area compared with average wages in all areas.

In calculating the average per diem routine operating cost for a given group of hospitals, hospitals with significant understaffing problems or that otherwise experience significant cost differentials resulting from failure to fully meet the standards of participation in the Medicare and Medicaid programs are to be excluded. Any hospital so excluded from the calculation of the group average shall receive the lesser of (1) actual costs or (2) the reimbursement limit for its appropriate group. The intent is to hold such institutions to the limit but not make the incentive payments available to them.

In an area where the wage level for hospitals is significantly higher than the general area wage level (relative to the relationship between hospital wages and general wages in other areas), the wage level for hospitals would be used instead of the general area wage level in calculating the fiscal 1979 per diem payment rate. In future years, area wage levels would be used.

To adjust for changes in the costs of the "mix of goods and services (including personnel and non-personnel costs) comprising routine operating costs," the hospital would be permitted to increase its payment rate in line with its costs, but by no more than the average percentage increase for hospitals in the area.[7] Adjustments will also be made to take account of unexpected changes in a hospital's classification.

The incentive reimbursement mechanism proposed by Senator Talmadge is intended to reward those hospitals that have costs less than the average for their category, but not to penalize those hospitals whose costs are higher than the average for their class so long as their costs are not in excess of 120 percent of the group's adjusted per diem payment rate. Specifically, a hospital that experiences per diem routine operating costs that are below the per diem payment rate established for that hospital would be reimbursed for its Medicare and Medicaid patients at a rate equal to its actual costs, plus an incentive payment equal to 50 percent of the difference between the group's payment rate and the actual cost, with a limit on the incentive payment equal to 5 percent of the group's payment rate. The hospital and the government thus share the benefits from cost savings when costs are below the established payment rate. When costs are in excess of the payment rate, the reimbursement would be for the greater of either (1) the actual costs, if those costs do not exceed 120 percent of the payment rate; or (2) a comparably defined amount if the hospital "had been classified in the bed-size category nearest to the category in which the hospital was actually classified, but not exceeding the hospital's actual routine operating costs."[8] This latter clause modifies the bed size categories slightly and permits the reimbursement to be somewhat greater than 120 percent of costs. It does limit the increases to actual costs within the specified upper limit.

This incentive mechanism is presumably based on the assumption that hospitals will be able to bring their costs down below the average by reducing inefficiency. This cost cutting would be more difficult for those hospitals that are efficient but have high costs for reasons such as their case mix than it would be for those hospitals that are inefficient. Those hospitals that are below the average for their group would have a natural advantage because they would be starting from a lower cost base. Thus, even if they experienced a very high rate of increase in costs, or became inefficient, they could still qualify for the incentive payment. Consequently, the bill provides these hospitals with windfall discretionary funds to spend. For example, a hospital with a case mix less complex than the average for the group in which it is classified may qualify for a bonus payment even if it is inefficient.

The concept of providing an incentive for reducing costs or for stemming the rate of cost increase is valid in principle. Interesting problems arise, however, as to the effectiveness of incentives in nonprofit organizations. A possible limitation is that there is no "owner" to receive rewards or to pay penalties. Incentives may have an effect if they help or hinder a hospital in achieving its goals, as determined by its administrators, trustees, and physicians.

A basic weakness of the proposal's incentive reimbursement is the formula proposed. A hospital that experiences costs higher than its group's rate is automatically reimbursed for costs in excess of this payment rate (subject to the 120 percent limit) and thus there seems to be little incentive for it to hold down costs. To rectify this weakness in the incentive reimbursement formula, the formula could be altered to provide penalties for those hospitals that have costs higher than the average for their group. The disadvantage of such an alteration is that it may cause greater hospital opposition to the proposal. The industry is likely to be more willing to accept classification when they benefit by an incentive payment for costs below the group average without being penalized for costs above the group average. If the classification system in the Talmadge bill could be made more sensitive, perhaps a comprehensive efficiency adjustment could be added.[9]

HOSPITAL CLASSIFICATION

The key to the functioning of the Talmadge proposal is the classification system to be developed by the Secretary. If the classification scheme is not realistic, the reimbursement formula can impose severe constraints on individual hospitals. The burden of the formula will be felt most by those hospitals that currently have costs well in excess of the average for the group in which they are placed. For this group of hospitals, the burden will be felt most by those hospitals that are relatively efficient, since they will have less flexibility to reduce costs. A classification system thus must be developed that takes into account warranted deviations in cost from the average of a group. The areawide wage rate adjustment is one step in this direction. The exclusion of certain types of costs—for example, energy costs, which are less comparable among hospitals across different areas—is another. A problem in making too many adjustments or in classifying hospitals into groups that are too small, however, is that it might create an inappropriate incentive for hospitals to take actions that change their category and create additional administrative burdens.

ADDITIONAL FEATURES

Another feature of the Talmadge proposal is an exemption for ancillary services. However, if a major cause of the rapid hospital inflation is an excessive rate of expansion in both hospital services and medical technology, this exemption will not constrain inflation. It may even contribute to it if it encourages hospitals to shift their expansion and growth objectives even more toward ancillary services. It also allows hospitals and third party payers to avoid facing the real issue of the cost-quality tradeoff associated with increased services.

The bill also exempts from coverage energy expenses and malpractice insurance costs. The rationale for excluding such costs is that, because these costs may not be comparable among hospitals and geographical areas, they would essentially confound a classification scheme. The costs associated with educational and training programs are exempt for similar reasons. Additionally exempted from the coverage under the per diem payment rate is the cost of "non-administration physicians." One recent trend in hospitals is the expansion of their salaried medical staff. While this increases hospital-billed costs, it would most likely not involve a substantial net increase in health care costs, because fee for service billings would be correspondingly reduced. The danger in this exemption is that hospitals may attempt to allocate additional resources to their salaried medical staff in excess of the amount needed to provide the level of care required. The motivation for such action would be the same as that for the expansion of any service, since an expanded medical staff adds prestige to the hospital.

In its present form, the Talmadge proposal does not provide a reimbursement formula for all components of hospital costs. For those components that are not included in the "routine operating costs" category, the bill states:

> The Secretary shall, at the earliest practical date, develop additional methods for reimbursing hospitals for all other costs, ... Those methods shall provide appropriate classification and reimbursement systems designed to ordinarily permit comparisons of the cost centers . . . similar in terms of size and scale of operation, prevailing wage levels, nature, extent, and appropriate volume of the services furnished, and other factors which have a substantial impact on hospital costs.[10]

This provision clearly has the intent of providing the information needed to monitor more closely the actual ancillary service costs incurred in a hospital, in order to determine if there have been unwarranted increases in these costs. The data collected would provide an information base for including additional categories of costs within the reimbursement program.

Another difficulty with the Talmadge formula is that the payment rate is to be on a per diem basis. With any per diem rate, a hospital can affect its total payments by adjusting its length of stay. To illustrate the type of effect that could be observed, consider a hospital that finds that it is at the high cost end of the group in which it is classified. To qualify for the incentive payment, the hospital could increase its average length of stay by not discharging patients as early as it otherwise would have. Since the last day of a stay is typically less costly than an earlier day, the cost of the last or incremental day is likely to be below the average cost and, hence, below the payment rate. Increases in the length of stay thus would decrease the hospital's average per diem cost, consequently increasing the safety margin between its actual routine cost per diem and the 120 percent limit. This behavior would increase total reimbursement by an amount greater than the marginal cost of the added day while at the same time decreasing the risk of exceeding the 120 percent group "cap." If the increase in patient days reduced the average cost per diem sufficiently, a high cost hospital could even qualify for an incentive payment.

To avoid this type of manipulation, the bill contains a paragraph that states:

> Where the Secretary finds that a hospital has manipulated its patient mix, or patient flow, or provides less than the normal range and extent of patient service, or where an unusually large proportion of routine nursing service is provided by private-duty nurses, the routine operating costs of that hospital shall be deemed equal to whichever is less: the amount determined without regard to this subsection, or the amount determined under subparagraph (B) [The reimbursement formula].[11]

To monitor "manipulation," a detailed and uniform cost-reporting system is necessary, although it may impose additional costs on hospitals to the extent that hospitals must revise their current procedures. The desirability of instituting a uniform accounting system is considered in Chapter 6.

The Talmadge bill will determine the per diem payment rates based on fiscal 1978 costs. This basis provides the hospital industry an incentive to increase costs during that year in order to have a margin within which it can operate in the following years. The administration's bill seeks to avoid this problem by using prelegislation periods as the base for determining allowable rates. This issue will be discussed in more detail in Chapter 6.

An important feature of the Talmadge bill, not contained in the administration's proposal, is that it allows for exemptions in the payment rate for costs associated with severance pay, mothballing, and other expenses related to the reduction in beds. These transitional allowances for terminated beds will be limited to no more than fifty hospitals during the first two years of the plan.

An additional feature of the proposed legislation is that the designated planning agency must approve any capital expenditure in excess of $100,000, as a condition to Medicare and Medicaid reimbursement for capital and direct operating costs associated with those expenditures. If the planning agencies are effective in determining the benefits of a proposed capital expenditure, this provision could have a significant effect on the rate of increase in hospital costs. There is, however, considerable skepticism about the ability of planning agencies to make such evaluations effectively.

Chapter 6

General Components of Cost Containment Alternatives

This chapter presents analyses of those components of cost containment alternatives that are included in both the administration and the Talmadge proposals and that would be likely to be included in any other proposal. The issues considered are (1) classification procedures and the measurement of hospital output, (2) anticipation effects, and (3) uniform accounting systems.

CLASSIFICATION AND THE DEFINITION OF OUTPUT

In order to compare costs across hospitals or to compare costs for an individual hospital over time, the similarity of the outputs being produced must first be measured. It is evident, however, that hospitals produce a large number of different outputs and that the mix of outputs will affect hospital costs.

One approach to this comparison problem is to classify hospitals by the types of patients treated. The objective in this case would be to develop patient classes that take into account the wide variety of diagnoses, the variations in the degree of morbidity and disability for any disagnosis, the effect of multiple diagnoses, and a multitude of other patient characteristics that influence the utilization of hospital resources. The rationale for classification has been described by Thompson, Mross, and Fetter:

> We assume that the control of cost is inextricably linked with the processes of patient care in terms of resource use, and rests upon understanding

the patient management process as it is applied appropriately to unique classes of patients. It is not sufficient to deal with utilization review and quality of care as a process separable from the expenditure of manpower, facilities and equipment in delivering that care, or vice versa. Research is going forward to link these three elements of cost, utilization, and quality to form the basis for hospital comparisons needed for rate reviews and rate setting.

The critical need is for a method by which hospitals can be characterized in terms of the services they provide to patients and the resources consumed for each delivery incident. What is required is the ability to describe the unique patient care processes delivered by each hospital and to measure the costs incurred in producing this mix of services for patient care.

With this approach, a state or region will be able to implement equitable rate setting, monitor hospital performance, and at the same time produce and feed back to each hospital the information it needs to review and evaluate its own performance and quality criteria.[1]

While this approach is a logical way of treating the effect of inter-hospital differences in the type of output produced, the difficulty in working at the level of patient classes has led to research whose purpose is to develop classification systems for hospitals as a whole instead of for patient groups. The objective is to group hospitals that are producing essentially the same mix and level of output or services. Having thus classified hospitals, it would then be possible to evaluate the performance of each member within a group. Payment can then be made on the basis of group experience, adjusted in part for individual experience.

Performance under such legislation will depend importantly on how well this grouping can be performed. While there are many variables that can be used in the classification procedure, the objective in all cases is to use characteristics that represent the "type of output" produced by each hospital.

A variety of statistical methods have been used to develop hospital classification systems, and the criteria by which these classification procedures should be evaluated are: first, the choice of characteristics on which the classification rests should be based on an understanding of the factors that determine the type of hospital output.[2] Second, the measure of similarity must differentiate hospitals that produce different products. Third, the particular statistical method used should capture the structural relationship between hospital characteristics and type of output. In addition, the procedure should be viewed by hospital administrators as equitable and well designed. It should be highly resolute, producing clear-cut categories with few exceptional cases, and it should be reasonably easy to administer.

Finally, the characteristics used should not be easily manipulable by hospitals for their own purposes. It should come as no surprise that no current method satisfies all these criteria and that our ability to classify hospitals in a satisfactory manner is limited. A classification scheme that is too detailed, however, essentially treats each hospital as unique and thus deserving of special, individualized treatment.

An additional problem associated with the use of classification systems is the identification of the source of the remaining "within group" variation in cost. If it were assumed that such within group variation in cost is caused by variation in efficiency, then an objective would be to identify this inefficiency so that the incentives in the cost containment program could lead to its reduction. The Talmadge proposal would determine the per diem payment rate for routine operating costs as the average per diem routine operating costs for the category in which the hospital is expected to be classified (with an area adjustment for the labor cost component). Thus, all within group differences from the average would be treated as variations in efficiency. In Chapter 3, it was suggested that technical inefficiency is not likely to be substantial in any given hospital and that to proceed as if it were would penalize the efficient but high cost hospitals within the group (due to unidentified differences in case mix, for example). As stated before, such hospitals would have the greatest difficulty in reducing costs to the group average.

If, on the other hand, it is assumed that, for the most part, the within group variation in cost is associated with the remaining variation in the type of output produced, the policy must deal specifically with whether the type of output is appropriate given the needs of the community and the availability of financial resources.

CONTROLS AND ANTICIPATION EFFECTS

In applying any form of control, one must deal with the problem of industry anticipation. If hospitals anticipate that controls will be introduced, they could take actions now that would ultimately weaken the impact of the controls. Attention has already been directed at this issue in connection with our discussion of specific provisions of the administration and the Talmadge bills.

In order to explore the issues of fairness and effectiveness more generally, we will consider the anticipatory behavior of the hospital industry. Individual hospitals have certainly been aware of public dissatisfaction with rising costs and the possibility of government intervention. It is surely possible that some hospitals may already have taken actions to reduce their vulnerability if cost or capital controls were imposed. Suppose, for example, that a hospital predicts that two years from now it would not be permitted to expand its facilities through capital investment. Any facilities that seemed desirable for the long-term plan of the hospital, given the projected costs of capital fundraising, would most likely be started within the two years. Therefore, within the two years, operating costs would have risen prematurely, and the proposed restrictions on capital spending would be challenged on the basis of unfinished work in progress. Moreover, limits on increases in operating costs would appear to be particularly harmful to such an institution insofar as the institution has put itself in the situation in which uniform controls would appear to be "unfair."

The point of this illustration is that if the cost containment program and its exceptions for "fairness" have been anticipated correctly, anticipatory behavior will largely frustrate the short-run impact of the program. Hospitals that did not anticipate fairness exemptions for increased operating cost due to capital expansion in progress will have engaged in less expansion and will not qualify for the fairness exemptions. The first general proposition that is suggested by this analysis is that regulatory proposals that constrain future behavior, but endorse the legitimacy of all past behavior and attempt to be "fair" in reducing the impact on those most adversely affected, will lead to two undesirable consequences: (1) hospital anticipation of this type of regulation will tend to reduce the effect of regulation on the social objective and (2) hospitals that believe they cannot offset the future impact of regulation will be permanently at a competitive disadvantage relative to hospitals that successfully frustrated the objectives of the program.

One basic implication of this general proposition is that a regulatory proposal for cost containment should be contemplated only as a long-term policy, so that the effect of the preemptive strategic behavior will be overshadowed by later years of effective regulation. A second implication is that a transitional program will guide the anticipations of the industry about future programs, tending to promote strategic behavior that could frustrate similar legislation in the future.

UNIFORM ACCOUNTING
AND REPORTING SYSTEMS

In order to implement the administration's or the Talmadge cost control procedures, monitoring and reimbursement procedures are required both for ex ante payment rate determination and for ex post settlement. The conventional approach to monitoring and reimbursement is to use accounting procedures for allocating fixed and joint costs among cost centers or other organizational units. While economic theory indicates that no purpose, either of resource allocation or pricing, can be served by such allocation, such accounting procedures are nevertheless used in order to set payment rates that are intended to produce revenue equal to the sum of fixed and variable costs. Such an accounting procedure designed to develop reimbursable costs will not necessarily yield the information required for good management of the institution.

The need for accounting information is multidimensional, and no one system can serve all purposes adequately. Hospitals will surely want to maintain additional accounting and information systems to promote effectiveness of management. However, it is important that those accounts used to determine costs for purpose of reimbursement be constructed according to uniform principles. Otherwise, if hospitals are permitted flexibility in these accounts, they could manipulate the cost allocation procedures. When a provider wishes to change its allocation basis for a particular cost center, or the order in which the cost centers are allocated, obtaining approval of the fiscal intermediary or third party payer should be required.

Accounting approaches to rate setting are firmly entrenched. In all likelihood, they are the only approaches that can realistically be expected to be used by hospitals, third party payers, and government agencies. The accounting approaches are based on identifying directly assignable costs, primarily short-run variable costs plus some fixed costs, and then allocating common costs on some arbitrary but "reasonable" basis. Since the allocations are arbitrary, hospitals have considerable flexibility in determining the "costs" on which rates are to be based. To monitor compliance with a national program, a uniform allocation procedure is desirable. Such a uniform procedure is particularly necessary in conjunction with either the administration or the Talmadge proposals, because they both exempt certain types of services from controls. In the administration proposal, for example, outpatient services are exempt, so one immediate way in which hospitals can reduce their "costs subject to control" is to allocate a greater amount of the common costs to outpatient services. Such reallocations, which are certainly in the interests of the hospital, would reduce the effectiveness of the controls. Similarly, in the Talmadge proposal, since ancillary services are exempt, "routine operating costs" can be "reduced" by allocating a greater amount of common costs to ancillary services. The remainder of this section is devoted to more detailed examination of the desirability of a uniform accounting system.

In testimony on HR 6575, the American Hospital Association expressed official opposition to HR 4211 that is now part of Section 19 of HR 3. HR 6575 establishes a uniform functional accounting system. The AHA stated: "We were very concerned that under the bill a uniform functional accounting system would be mandated for hospitals without exception."[3]

Under HR 6575, a uniform functional accounting and statistical system for health services institutions would include:

1. Uniform accounting practices;
2. A uniform functional chart of accounts, including definitions of specific accounts and (as appropriate) subaccounts, a uniform numerical coding system of such accounts and subaccounts, and a uniform classification of expenses within such accounts;
3. Uniform statistical measures of productivity;
4. Uniform methods and statistical measures for cost accounting and cost allocations among accounts;
5. A uniform cost and statistical reporting system; and
6. A uniform discharge abstract and uniform billing system.

Why might hospitals oppose the uniform functional accounting system proposal? One answer is that HR 6575 removes the flexibility in classification of accounting cost and choice in application of accounting methods. This in turn directly affects hospital management's ability to allocate cost to areas within the hospital that could increase cost reimbursement. In addition, there may be justifiable "special circumstances" that cannot be accommodated by a uniform procedure. To deal with the last objection, however, an exceptions process might be more suitable.

The uniform accounting system would reduce the freedom of allocation now available under the current system of cost contract reimbursement. It is difficult to predict what the exact form the law would take if enacted. However, if only one method of allocation were allowed, if the allocation bases were predetermined (i.e., a unique set were selected in advance), and if a procedure for classification of expenses into predetermined cost pools or functional accounts were established, then there would exist one unique manner to determine a hospital's reimbursement amount under Medicare and Medicaid cost contracts. If this method were employed for cost determination for all third party cost contracts, then alteration of the accounting system would not be available to a hospital to maximize reimbursement.

The administration's proposal does not remove the flexibility permitted under the current system and therefore does not prevent changes in allocation bases that would allocate a greater share of cost to outpatient services, for example, since they are exempt from the revenue limit. The Talmadge proposal, while calling for the uniform functional accounting system, regulates only routine operating cost. Costs associated with capital, education and training programs, malpractice insurance, and so forth would continue, at least initially, to be reimbursed under current laws. It should be noted that even though the uniform functional accounting system may be adopted, it may not lead to a unique set of allocations since the federal regulations may be open to many interpretations.

✳

Appendixes

Appendix A

American Hospital Association Index of Hospital Input Prices 1974–1975

Components of American Hospital Association Index of Hospital Input Prices, 1974–75.

Component	Percent Weight	1974	1975	Percent Change	All Items Less Component Percent Change
All Items	100.00	157.1	189.7	20.75	22.70
Administration and General	13.36	138.4	149.6	8.1	
Communications	2.68	131.5	135.6	3.1	21.24
Telephone	2.13	121.4	125.3	3.2	21.13
Postal Charges	0.55	170.5	175.4	2.9	20.85
Audit, Accounting and Miscellaneous Services	2.68	152.0	166.6	9.6	21.06
Travel	0.92	137.7	150.6	9.4	20.86
Other	7.07	136.1	148.5	9.1	21.64
Insurance (excluding Workmen's Compensation)	2.37	396.5	1123.4	183.3	16.81
Malpractice	1.62	522.5	1582.7	202.9	17.75
Property	0.75	124.2	131.4	5.8	20.86
Dietary	11.89	161.7	175.4	8.5	22.40
Household and Maintenance	14.02	171.5	199.9	16.6	21.43
Housekeeping	1.82	141.9	177.4	25.0	20.67
Soaps and Detergents	1.21	133.6	161.9	21.2	20.75
Other	0.61	158.3	208.0	31.4	20.69
Laundry	3.38	149.5	163.6	9.4	21.15
Flatwork	1.36	170.1	187.3	10.1	20.90
Sheets	2.02	135.6	147.6	8.8	21.00

Component	Percent Weight	1974	1975	Percent Change	All Items Less Component Percent Change
Household and Maintenance (cont'd.)					
Maintenance of Personnel	0.58	136.1	148.5	9.1	20.80
Operation of Plant	6.32	194.8	234.0	20.1	20.80
Electricity	2.22	152.8	175.4	14.8	20.89
Natural Gas	1.90	154.6	215.3	39.3	20.39
Fuel Oil No. 6	1.70	272.0	309.4	13.8	20.87
Fuel Oil No. 4	0.38	272.0	309.4	13.8	20.78
Fuel Oil No. 2	0.12	272.0	309.4	13.8	20.76
Repairs	1.93	171.6	187.6	9.3	20.98
Professional Service Cost					
(*Nonsalary*)	43.94	144.5	158.6	9.8	29.33
Drugs	7.47	112.7	126.6	12.3	21.43
Medical Supplies	25.48	151.4	165.6	9.4	24.63
Medical Records	1.76	136.1	148.5	9.1	20.96
Laboratory	9.23	152.6	167.1	9.5	21.90
Medical Supplies	4.62	151.4	165.6	9.4	21.30
Rental SMA–12 and Reagents	4.15	152.0	166.6	9.6	21.23
Maintenance and Repair	0.46	171.6	187.6	9.3	20.80
Capital Expense	14.43	155.8	170.2	9.2	22.70
Fixed Capital	6.49	176.6	197.8	12.0	21.36
Movable Capital	3.61	137.7	154.2	12.0	21.08
Interest	4.33	140.2	142.1	1.4	21.63

Source: American Hospital Association, (unpublished data based on Panel Surveys, courtesy of Dr. David Drake).

Appendix B

A Policy Analysis of the Expanded Talmadge Proposal

Expanded Version of S 1470 Developed by
Senate Finance Committee Staff

The expanded Talmadge proposal represents a significant change from the initial version. First, it adds to the incentive payments for Medicare and Medicaid patients a system of annual limits that apply to hospital inpatient care revenues from all payers. Second, these limits cover revenues from routine services and ancillary services. Third, the revenue limits would be applied to hospitals' accounting periods that begin on or after July 1, 1978 (in the case of routine services) and July 1, 1979 (in the case of ancillary services).

Separate revenue limits would be calculated for the hospital's routine services (bed, board, routine nursing, and supplies, etc.) and for its ancillary services (X-rays, laboratory tests, drugs, etc.). It should be recognized that the accounting procedures needed to make this separation are somewhat arbitrary. If each institution were allowed to define its own procedures, it would be in a position to manipulate the separation of costs to its benefit. However, if, as has been suggested by health staff members of the Senate Finance Committee, the separation is based on a uniform set of weights for allocating common costs, these weights would at best represent an accurate separation for some "average" institution, but would be increasingly inappropriate for hospitals less and less like the average.

The reason for separate limits for routine services and ancillary services is the desire to use different methods to calculate each of the two limits. The method for calculating the routine service revenue limits requires the comparison of routine service costs of similar hospitals by (1) grouping hospitals, (2) computing an average routine service revenue per diem for each group, and (3) then comparing the per diem revenue of each hospital within the group to the group average. The maximum per diem routine service revenue limit for the hospital's first annual accounting period would be equal to 120 percent of the group average. The routine service revenue for the second and subsequent years of the program would be increased by 103 percent of the estimated increase in the group average routine costs over the previous year. The maximum routine per diem service revenue limit would be multiplied by the total number of days of hospital care provided in the year to determine the hospital's total revenue limit from routine services.

RATIONALE FOR THE REVENUE LIMITS

This method recognizes that there are differences among hospitals that may lead to differences in efficient cost levels. It also recognizes that some of the variation in costs is due in part to variations in efficiency among hospitals and that cost containment should place more direct constraints on high cost (presumably inefficient) hospitals than on low cost (presumably efficient) ones. In order to affect costs in these relatively low cost hospitals as well, the Talmadge proposal also provides for incentive payments under federal programs for those hospitals with routine costs below the average for their group. For patients covered by Medicare and Medicaid, such hospitals would receive their actual costs plus one-half of the difference between actual costs and the average for their group. As noted in our discussion of the earlier Talmadge proposal, this type of incentive mechanism appears to be based on the assumption that hospitals will respond by trying to lower their costs below the group average in order to increase net revenues through reductions in inefficiency. Proponents feel that the attractiveness of "free money" will elicit the desired result. However, reductions in costs would require a larger sacrifice of service intensity for those hospitals that are already efficient but have high costs for reasons not accounted for by the classification scheme (such as their case mix) than would be required for those hospitals that are inefficient. The mechanism could also reward some inefficient hospitals—those hospitals that are inefficient but have costs below the group average for reasons not considered by the classification scheme.

Compared to the administration's proposed revenue limits, the revised Talmadge limits would in general be much less constraining. An "average" hospital—that is, one with routine per diem costs equal to the average of its group—could increase its revenues from routine care by as much as 20 percent in the first year. In subsequent years it could then only increase its revenues by 3 percent per year more than the increase in input prices, but the difference between the 20 percent increase permitted in the Talmadge proposal and the 9 percent figure permitted in the administration bill, even if spread over several years, is not negligible.

Moreover, the proposal also provides an exception for a hospital that can demonstrate that its routine costs exceed the limit because of (1) underutilization of beds or facilities where such beds or facilities are necessary to meet the needs of an underserved area, or (2) an unusual patient mix that results in a greater intensity of routine care. We might well expect that those institutions that are affected by the 120 percent limit will apply for such an exception. Because part of the variation in costs within groups is likely to be associated with legitimate variation in the case mix or the nature (intensity) of the services produced, it may well be difficult to reject these applications on objective grounds. In short, it would appear that the routine service limit is unlikely to be an effective cost containment strategy. The variation in costs arising from "inefficiencies" is very unlikely to exceed 20 percent of the average for the great majority of hospitals.

ANCILLARY SERVICES REVENUE LIMIT

The coverage of ancillary services in the present proposal overcomes a serious deficiency in the previous Talmadge proposal. If major causes of rapid hospital inflation are excessive rates both of the expansion of hospital services and of the acquisition of medical technology, coverage of ancillary services is essential for the success of a cost containment program.

The expanded Talmadge proposal applies the administration's general approach to setting limits on ancillary service revenues, on an interim basis, until a more permanent solution can be developed. Ancillary service revenues would be limited to a rate of growth that takes account of changes in general wage levels in the hospital's locality and national changes in the prices that hospitals pay for equipment, supplies, and other goods used in the production of care. To determine this limit, ancillary costs would be separated into two components, a portion attributed to labor costs and a portion attributed to the purchase cost of nonlabor inputs. In addition, adjustment would be made to accommodate approved expansion in patient care services. Operating costs associated with approved capital expansion would be passed through, and a fixed percentage increase of 1 percent would be granted to accommodate all other intensity increases for which no approval process currently exists.

If the prices that hospitals pay for the labor and nonlabor factors of production are increasing at the rate of the GNP deflator, then with only a 1 percent intensity allowance, the ancillary service revenue limit in the Talmadge proposal would grow at a lower rate than in the administration's proposal.[1] However, since the GNP deflator has been increasing in recent years at a lower rate than indexes of hospital nonlabor inputs, the apparently more stringent intensity limitation on the percentage increase in revenues in the Talmadge proposal might be partially or completely offset.

The expanded Talmadge proposal also provides that "if a given hospital's revenue exceeded only one of the two limits, the excess revenues could be reduced to the extent they fell below the other limit."[2] What this means is that a hospital can exceed the ancillary services revenue limit by the amount they are below the routine service revenue limit. It is not clear how this would affect the potential incentive payment; but in light of the apparent laxness of the routine service revenue limit, it clearly does weaken the limit on ancillary service revenue.

RESOLUTION OF
CONFLICTING APPROACHES

The concerns that motivated the expanded version of the Talmadge proposal can, to some extent, be incorporated into the administration's proposal in a way that would produce an improved program. We discuss such a combination in connection with a number of specific topics.

Permanent versus Temporary Program

The administration has proposed a transitional program without defining the overall permanent structure within which the transition might be understood. There exists considerable concern about this lack of specification in light of the arbitrariness of the across the board revenue limits and the open-ended nature of the transition. An implication of our policy analysis is that a regulatory proposal for cost containment should be contemplated only as a long-term policy, so that the effects of preemptive strategic behavior will be overshadowed by later years of effective regulation. A second implication is that a transitional program will guide the anticipations of the industry about future programs, tending to promote strategic behavior that would frustrate similar legislation in the future.

There is need to recognize explicitly that some elements within a cost containment program must, of necessity, be arbitrary. Thus, emphasis should be placed on the *process* by which these elements can be equitably adjusted over time. Within a defined permanent structure, a transitional program could be very similar to the current administration proposal. Unresolved elements could then be further investigated by the Secretary within specific constraints.

Across the Board Limits versus Classification

The Talmadge proposal reflects a concern for individual differences among hospitals. In order to compare costs across hospitals or to compare costs for an individual hospital over time, the degree of similarity of the mix of outputs and of changes in that mix must be considered. An across the board limit on the rate of revenue growth would be insensitive to differences in the nature of the product produced. While this insensitivity might not be unfair over a short period of time, it could be serious if the across the board limits were applied for some longer period.

Limits on Costs versus Limits on Rates
of Revenue Growth

Our policy analysis concluded that the primary dimensions of the hospital cost inflation problem were the rapid increase in service intensity, inefficiency at the industry level, and the inability to make explicit cost-quality tradeoffs. These conclusions imply that, for the most part, the variation across hospitals in hospital costs is associated with variation in the types of output produced and that policy must deal specifically with whether the types of output are appropriate to the needs of the community and the availability of resources. At the same time, some are concerned that part of the variation in unit cost is caused by variation in efficiency and that an objective of a cost containment program should be to design incentives to lead to its reduction. However, while variation across institutions in levels of efficiency is one possible source of variation in unit costs, variation in efficiency cannot adequately explain the continuing excessive rates of cost inflation; there is no reason to suppose that inefficiency has been increasing at a rapid rate, if at all. Any explanation of the cost inflation must also include the effect of industry- or systemwide inefficiency.

The level of inefficiency of the individual hospital is the target of the Talmadge proposal for dealing with routine operating costs. However, as we have discussed above, the incentives for efficiency contained in the Talmadge procedure are not as compelling as might be desired, and the limits in revenue are not likely to constrain most hospitals.

The administration's proposal established a limit for each hospital that does not depend on its own behavior or characteristics, whereas the Talmadge proposal is concerned with the relation of an individual hospital's costs to average costs of a group of similar hospitals. It would be possible to make the administration's revenue increase limit also depend on deviations from levels of group performance by the inclusion of a "comprehensive efficiency adjustment." For example, let the national revenue limit be *NR* percent. This might be equal to the sum of the increase in an index of prices that hospitals pay for labor and nonlabor inputs plus an explicit allowance for increases in intensity and expansion of service equal to the real growth in GNP. Now consider a group of similar hospitals. For these hospitals, we can calculate the group average cost per adjusted admission, $\bar{c}$. Then if a particular hospital has an average cost per adjusted admission equal to c, we can determine that hospital's revenue limit according to the formula

$$R = NR + \propto \frac{(\bar{c}-c)}{\bar{c}} \times 100$$

That is, if a hospital's average cost per adjusted admission is 10 percent below the group average, its revenue limit would be 1 percent above the national revenue limit (assuming $\propto = 0.1$). Similarly, if a hospital's average cost per adjusted admission is 20 percent above the group average, its revenue limit would be 2 percent below the national revenue limit.

A TRANSITIONAL PROGRAM

In the long run, we prefer a hospital cost containment program with more discretion in the allocations of a national revenue limit than is contained in an efficiency adjustment. Such a program, built upon the national health planning and development system is described in Part I of this volume. In the short run, it would be difficult to implement an efficiency adjustment based upon a hospital classification system; such classification systems are currently in an underdeveloped state. Thus, it would appear appropriate to consider the administration's proposal as the first stage of a transition that would involve the use of efficiency adjustments when a workable classification system was developed and, at a time when the national health planning system was more fully developed, a program of local discretion within the framework of national limits.

CLASSIFICATION SYSTEMS

The use of the "efficiency adjustment" or, for that matter, the Talmadge proposal for determining the routine service revenue limit requires that hospitals that are producing essentially the same level and mix of outputs or services be grouped. While there are many variables that can be used in the classification procedure, the objective in all cases is to use characteristics that represent the "type of output" produced by each hospital. The criteria by which the classification procedure should be evaluated have been described in preceding analysis (see pages 13 and 107).

As an example of the state of knowledge of classification systems, Phillip and Iyer have developed a community hospital classification system based on "product characteristic" variables, such as total number of facilities or services, teaching status, and variables designed to serve as proxies for the complexity of the institution's care and "external characteristics" variables such as the average per capita income in the county in which the hospital is located.[3] The procedure involves initial stratification by number of hospital beds and, within stratification, classification on the basis of cluster analysis. The technique of cluster analysis can be useful in attempting to discover a partition of hospitals. Each hospital is described by the characteristics of its product and its location, and the procedure identifies groups of hospitals with a similar configuration of characteristics.

In order to implement the cluster analysis, a measure of similarity must also be defined. Ideally, a measure should assure that two hospitals will be close when each is producing essentially the same type of care. Only if this is true can cost comparisons among the hospitals within a group be made with confidence. Of course, the variation in hospitals by type of output is more likely to be continuous, and thus, clear-cut groups of hospitals are unlikely to emerge from a clustering analysis. In establishing groups, it will be necessary to deal with a tradeoff between the objective of within group similarity and the objective that all hospitals be classifiable in a manageable number of groups. In achieving the latter objective, there will be, of necessity, some variation in type of output remaining within groups, and thus, some of the resulting within group cost variation must be recognized as legitimate.

Table B—1 presents a summary of the Phillip and Iyer groupings. The authors recognize the difficulty of the classification task, and they warn against the use of their system in a cost control system. They obtain seventy-one hospital groups with an average size of sixty-four hospitals. Four groups contained fewer than fifteen hospitals while eleven groups contained fewer than twenty hospitals. It also should be noted that considerable variation remains within groups.

The author's identification of "nonclusterable isolates" draws attention to the need for treating atypical hospitals through an exception process. These 484 nonclusterable isolates are "hospitals whose characteristics were so atypical that they could not be assigned to any cluster" given the procedures used for classification. It is questionable if a procedure that produces seventy-one groups with 5 to 239 members per group and defines 484 of 5,034 hospitals as unclassifiable is suitable for use in a cost containment program.

Given the present state of knowledge, the ability to classify hospitals in a satisfactory manner is limited, but classifying hospitals on the basis of characteristics known to affect efficient cost levels is better than treating them as if they were identical. A classification scheme that is too detailed, however, essentially treats each hospital as unique and thus deserving of special treatment.

VOLUME ADJUSTMENTS

The routine services revenue limit (at 120 percent of the group average per diem) increases in proportion to the increase in patient days. The volume adjustments for ancillary services are more complicated and are quite different from those in the administration's proposal. Suppose, to make things comparable, that average length of stay does

Table B—1. Number of Clusters of Hospitals and Nonclusterable Isolates by Stratum.

Stratum	Number of Licensed Beds	Number of Hospitals	Number of Clusters	Number of Inclusterable Isolates
I	6–49	1,378	16	110
II	50–99	1,271	22	85
III	100–299	1,666	22	177
IV	300–499	508	5	62
V	500+	211	6	50

Source: Data calculated from P.J. Phillip and R.N. Iyer, "Classification of Community Hospitals" *Health Services Research*, Winter, 1975, Vol. 10, No. 4; 349–368.

not change. Then a hospital whose admissions and patient days increased by 2 percent would be permitted a zero revenue increase under the administration's proposal, but a 2 percent increase under the expanded Talmadge proposal. In effect, the administration's proposal assumes that the additional (marginal) cost of small changes in output is zero, while the Talmadge proposal assumes that marginal cost equals average costs, so that costs rise proportionately. For larger output changes, the administration and the Talmadge proposals both permit revenues to rise by half of the increase in volume. The expanded Talmadge proposal is also more generous for those institutions whose volume is falling. In fact, if admissions fall below 90 percent of the base period, the revenue limit will decline at a marginal rate of 50 percent of the allowed revenue per admission regardless of the size of the revenue decrease. In the administration's proposal, the revenue limit declined by 100 percent of the allowed revenue per admission for decreases of more than 15 percent in admissions.

As we have discussed earlier, if either program is viewed as permanent, the relevant marginal cost to be considered is the long-run marginal cost, and this cost may be much greater than the zero implied by the administration's proposal. It is also likely to be somewhat less than the average cost implied by the Talmadge proposal, although the latter may be closer to the truth.

If, however, changes in the volume of days of stay come about in part by changes in length of stay, then the revised Talmadge proposal almost surely permits hospitals to be overcompensated for routine costs. The cost of the resources consumed during a patient's last few days of stay, over the resources for routine care, is surely less than the average. The patient requires less nursing time, may have less of a requirement for a special diet, and so forth. Moreover, since routine cost per day can be reduced by increasing stays, the Talmadge proposal would provide an incentive to hospitals to do so. Ideally, routine costs volume adjustments should depend both on changes in admissions and on changes in days of stay (or of stay per admission); at a minimum, changes in length of stay should be incorporated into the volume adjustment formula.

EXCLUDED CATEGORIES OF COST

The routine services revenue limit would not apply to revenues attributable to capital related costs; costs of education and training programs; costs of interns', residents' and physicians' medical services; energy costs of heating and cooling; certain costs unique to proprietary institutions; and malpractice insurance costs. The exemption of specific cost categories with provisions to pass excessive cost increases through to the revenue limit clearly removes the incentive to contain costs within that category. Since levels of costs in the categories exempted are likely not to be comparable among hospitals, their exemption in calculating the routine services revenue limit becomes almost a necessity. If, as we have suggested, these levels are used only to determine an "efficiency adjustment" to the revenue increase limit, their exemption is not serious. The implication is that their inclusion would confound an efficiency comparison among hospitals in terms of routine services costs per diem.

TECHNICAL REQUIREMENTS
OF THE TALMADGE PROPOSAL

There are three broad areas in which the revised Talmadge proposal appears to have technical requirements in excess of what is presently known.

First, the allocation of costs into routine and ancillary categories requires some method that is uniform across hospitals, appropriate for individual hospitals, and feasible to implement. In particular, no mutually satisfactory method to allocate those costs that are specific to either type of activity, and to distribute common costs over outputs, exists. The establishment of a system of accounting and uniform functional cost reporting does not, by its mere existence or mandated use, insure comparability of cost among hospitals. While each hospital may be aggregating and allocating cost in the same manner and reporting the results in accordance with a uniform functional chart of accounts, comparability of results is not insured. The functional reporting categories may be the results of different technologies or of different vectors of services. Furthermore, historical cost allocation to individual functional areas results in a comingling of costs from different periods of time.

Second, fully acceptable wage and nonlabor input price indexes for the two components of ancillary costs have yet to be developed. In part, the development of such indexes and the classes of hospitals to which they should apply is a feasible but time-consuming empirical task. As discussed earlier, however, to the extent that such indexes measure prices of inputs purchased primarily by hospitals in noncompetitive markets, their use may enhance the monopsony power of input suppliers.

Third, the choice of the maximum range for routine costs per diem (120 percent or some other number) appears to be highly arbi-

Figure B-1. Hypothetical Distribution of Costs Per Diem for Hospitals Within a Group.

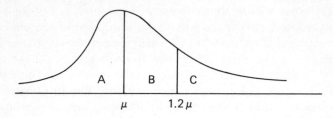

trary. Other than documenting the number of hospitals that would or would not be constrained by various limits and various grouping procedures, it is not obvious how one would go about choosing the "right" levels for the range. Furthermore, under the expanded Talmadge proposal, it would be possible with incentive payments to entail higher costs to the government, depending upon the distribution of costs within the group. Consider the distribution of costs per diem for "similar" hospitals within a particular group as shown in Figure B-1. Hospitals (in A) with costs per diem less than the group average, μ, receive positive incentive payments. Hospitals (in B) with costs per diem greater than the group average but less than 20 percent above the group average are fully reimbursed for their costs. Finally, hospitals (in C) with costs more than 20 percent above the group average receive a negative incentive (i.e., are penalized). If positive incentive payments are greater than disallowed costs in Group C, the government's cost may rise. This would certainly be the case if all hospitals had costs less than 20 percent above the group average, since there woule be positive incentive payments without savings.

CONCLUSION

The expanded Talmadge proposal may have a greater effect on containing costs than its original version. Some aspects of the new proposal could usefully be incorporated into the administration's program to provide a transitional stage to a more permanent program.

Appendix C

The Rogers and Rostenkowski Amendments to HR 6575

Both the Subcommittee on Health and the Environment of the House Interstate and Foreign Commerce Committee (Paul Rogers, Chairman) and the Subcommittee on Health of the Committee on Ways and Means (Dan Rostenkowski, Chairman) have proposed several changes in the administration's proposal. In this appendix, we will comment on some of those proposed changes. Other changes, which are of an administrative nature or which do not deal directly with the problem of hospital cost containment, will not be considered here.

SUBCOMMITTEE ON HEALTH AND THE ENVIRONMENT OF THE HOUSE INTERSTATE AND FOREIGN COMMERCE COMMITTEE—AMENDMENTS

Changes in the Formula for Cost Increases

The Rogers' subcommittee substituted a simpler formula for the administration's formula described in Chapter 4. Under this formula, the allowed rate of hospital cost inflation would be just 1.5 times the rate of change in the GNP deflator. The subcommittee also asked for the development of a more hospital-specific input price index by the Secretary of HEW by early 1979 and sought a recommendation on the desirability of wage passthroughs for nonsupervisory employees by the same date.

Compared to the original administration formula, the proposed change would not bring the rate of increase in service intensity down

133

to zero over time, because it would always permit hospital revenues to increase by more than hospital input costs. It would therefore not necessarily lead to a reduction in the hospital share of a growing real GNP, one of the peculiar features of the administration's program.

The subcommittee's suggestion has peculiarities of its own, however. Basically, it ties the rate of growth in intensity to the inflation rate (either economywide, as measured by the GNP deflator, or hospital-specific) after 1979. This provision would tend to induce fluctuations in the rate of change in the share of GNP going to hospitals. If real GNP always changed at a constant rate, the share would tend to increase most rapidly in inflationary times and contract (or increase less rapidly) in periods of price stability. (Real GNP growth has tended to be mildly positively related to the inflation rate, so this latter outcome might not be observed.) There appears to be no rationale, however, for tying the permitted rate of increase in service intensity to such a moving target. Indeed, permitting hospital service intensity to increase most rapidly when the inflation rate is high would seem to be destabilizing, in the sense that it would permit hospitals to expand more rapidly when input prices were increasing rapidly, while permitting them to expand less rapidly when input prices were more stable.

Incentive Payments

The Rogers proposal would permit incentive payments as in the Talmadge bill. These payments would be equal to 50 percent of the difference between allowed revenue per admission and cost per admission, except that any surplus thus earned would have to be used for (1) covering outpatient department deficits, (2) retiring long-term debt, and (3) uses that the Secretary of HEW determined would not add to operating costs and would be in the public interest.

This provision ostensibly encourages incentive reimbursement schemes. In practice it would likely be more restrictive than the administration's proposal, however, because it really only restricts the schemes that could be offered. The administration's bill, on the other hand, by not forbidding anything, would implicitly permit any mutually agreeable incentive reimbursement scheme between third party and hospital.

Discontinuance of Facilities

The bill contains a Title III in which government payments for retraining costs and other expenses of hospital closure or facility discontinuance, up to $500,000 for closing an entire hospital, are proposed. Such a program would presumably facilitate a decertification and closure procedure. This title also provides a mild penalty (reduction of federal reimbursement of 5 percent) for those facilities that refuse to close when such a suggestion is made by the area planning agency.

SUBCOMMITTEE ON HEALTH OF THE HOUSE WAYS AND MEANS COMMITTEE—AMENDMENTS

Description of the Program

The major distinguishing feature of the Rostenkowski proposal is the establishment of the federal government's cost containment program as a fallback if voluntary efforts to control costs fail to meet or exceed certain specified targets. The bill also contains some regulations for hospital payments to nonsalaried physicians. The latter regulations will not be discussed here.

The voluntary program must meet the following targets:

Calendar 1978:   1977 inflation rates less 2 percent or 1.5 times the rate of growth in the GNP deflator, whichever is greater.

Calendar 1979 and after: 1977 inflation rates less 4 percent or 1.5 times the rate of growth in the GNP deflator, whichever is greater.

If the target is not achieved in any year, the federal program will take effect in the following calendar year and will run for at least four years. The maximum permitted increase under the federal fallback program is 1.5 times the rate of growth in the GNP deflator; the other provisions of the fallback program are similar to those in the administration's bill.

If the fallback program does go into effect, a hospital's base level of revenue is the level in the accounting year that is two years prior to the initiation of the program, increased to the year immediately preceding the program by the lesser of the rate of increase goal of the voluntary effort or the hospital's actual rate of increase. If the actual rate of increase were less than the rate of growth in the GNP deflator, the latter would be used instead.

The Problem of Anticipation

The mechanism by which individual hospitals would be induced to adhere to the voluntary goal is quite unclear. Since any individual hospital's behavior is unlikely to have an appreciable effect on whether or not the industry achieves its goal, the success of the voluntary effort will depend upon the extent to which moral suasion and peer group pressure can override "free rider" or noncooperative behavior. There might even be antitrust issues involved in an attempt to do so.

A danger is that individual hospitals may not only simply ignore the voluntary effort, but that they could also use the "period of grace" it entails to engage in anticipatory behavior, pushing up costs even faster in order to get desired facilities and services before the mandatory program became effective. The base year adjustment described above is an attempt to discourage such behavior, but it may not be fully effective in doing so. For instance, suppose a hospital had planned some increases in services over the next five years that would be prevented or delayed by the imposition of mandatory controls. It might, accordingly, consider starting some or all of these programs in the first year of the voluntary effort, even though doing so would push its rate of cost increase up to or above the voluntary target.

The base year adjustment contains a provision to discourage a hospital from doing so, however. If the mandatory program were to take effect, a hospital would be permitted to increase its base year revenues and costs only by the voluntary effort's target rate, not by its actual rate. Consequently, if the mandatory program were to take effect, the actual increase permitted in the first year of that program would be reduced to the extent that the increase in the preceding year exceeded the voluntary effort guideline. For example, if the voluntary effort had a target of 12 percent, a hospital's actual increase was 16 percent, and the first year mandatory limit was 9 percent, the hospital would actually be able to have an increase of only 5 percent in the first year of the program. This means that the voluntary effort is "voluntary" only in a limited sense. A hospital that exceeded the voluntary guideline would have that guideline imposed in a mandatory ex post facto manner if the mandatory program were activated. The program is "voluntary" in the sense that there can be "voluntary" donations for a church supper, but all diners will be billed for the cost of the meal if insufficient funds are collected.

To some extent, a hospital may be able to seek and receive an exception from this rule on the basis of unfinished work in progress. A more important problem is that a hospital that would otherwise have increased its costs by less than the industry maximum would have an incentive to move up to the industry maximum, in order to get into its base new programs it intended to institute at some future date. A hospital that would otherwise have increased its cost by more than the voluntary effort guidelines may be induced to cut back somewhat, but it would most likely cut back only to the guideline maximum if it were sure that the voluntary effort would fail.

In summary, it is likely that many hospitals would have an incentive, at best, to just meet and, at worst, to exceed, the voluntary effort guidelines. The combination of a voluntary effort and a federal standby program does, however, preserve hospital self-regulation for a while longer. In fact, the voluntary effort may be the last alternative to some form of regulatory cost control for the hospital industry. Accordingly, it would appear appropriate that the performance of the hospital industry under the voluntary effort become a primary research and evaluation target.

Notes

Chapter 1

1. *The Hospital Cost Index* and *The Hospital Intensity Index* (Chicago: American Hospital Association, Hospital Research Center, 1977).

2. A. Scitovsky and N. McCall, *Changes in the Costs of Treatments of Selected Illnesses*, NCHSR Research Digest Series, DHEW Publication No. HRA–77–3161, (Washington D.C., U.S. Department of Health, Education, and Welfare, July 1976).

3. Institute of Medicine, "Assessing Quality in Health Care: An Evaluation" (Washington, D.C.: National Academy of Sciences, November 1976).

4. P. Gertman, Personal Communication, June 1977.

5. *Congressional Record—House*, April 25, 1977, p. H–3527, Summary of HR 6575.

6. *Congressional Record—House*, April 25, 1977, p. H–3528, Summary of HR 6575.

7. *The 1975 AHA Guide to the Health Care Field*, Chicago: American Hospital Association.

8. *Congressional Record—House*, April 25, 1977, p. H–3529, Summary of HR 6575.

9. *Selected Hospital Cost Containment Proposals: Major Provisions* (Washington, D.C.: Committee on Finance, U.S. Senate, October 11, 1977), p. 3.

Chapter 2

1. *Hospital Regulation: Report of the Special Committee on the Regulatory Process* (Chicago: American Hospital Association, 1977).

2. Joseph Newhouse and Vincent Taylor, "A New Type of Hospital Insurance: A Proposal for an Experiment" (Santa Monica, CA.: Rand, October 1970).

3. Paul Ellwood and Walter McClure, "Health Delivery Reform" (Minneapolis: InterStudy, 1976).

Chapter 3

1. M. Feldstein and A. Taylor, "The Rapid Rise of Hospital Costs," Harvard Institute of Economic Research, Discussion Paper No. 531, 1977.

2. Victor R. Fuchs, "The Earnings of Allied Health Personnel: Are Health Workers Underpaid?" *Explorations in Economic Research* 3, no. 3 (Summer 1976): 408–32.

3. President's Hospital Cost Containment Proposal (HR 6575): Joint Hearings Before the Subcommittee on Health, Committee on Ways and Means and the Subcommittee on Health and the Environment, Committee on Interstate and Foreign Commerce, U.S. House of Representatives, 95th Cong., May 11, 12 and 13, 1977, p. 688.

4. Ibid., p. 597.

5. Ibid., p. 542.

6. *The Problem of Rising Health Care Costs* (Washington, D.C.: Government Printing Office, 1976), U.S. Council on Wage and Price Stability.

7. President's Hospital Cost Containment Proposal (HR 6575): Joint hearings Before the Subcommittee on Health, Committee on Ways and Means and the Subcommittee on Health and the Environment, Committee on Interstate and Foreign Commerce, U.S. House of Representatives, 95th Congress, May 11, 12, and 13, 1977.

8. Victor R. Fuchs, *Who Shall Live?* (New York: Basic Books, Inc., 1974), p. 60.

9. M.V. Pauly and T. Beazoglou, "Using Charges to Analyze Hospital Costs and Costliness" (Evanston, Ill.: Northwestern University, May 1976); and R.G. Evans, "Behavioral Cost Functions for Hospitals," *Canadian Journal of Economics*, May 1971, pp. 198–215.

10. Feldstein and Taylor.

11. M.A. Morehead; R.S. Donaldson; S. Sanderson; and F.E. Burt, *A Study of the Quality of Hospital Care Secured by a Sample of Teamster Family Members in New York City* (New York: Columbia University School of Public Health, 1964); K.N. Williams and R.H. Brook, "Foreign Medical Graduates and their Impact on the Quality of Medical Care in the United States," *Health and Society; the Milbank Quarterly* 53, no. 4 (Fall 1975); and Edward F.X. Hughes, "Board Certification and the Quality of Surgical Care: An Examination of the Issues," Center for Health Services and Policy Research, Working Paper No. 2, Northwestern University, March 1977.

12. B.C. Payne and T.F. Lyons, *Method of Evaluating and Improving Personal Medical Care Quality: Episodes of Illness Study* (Chicago: American Hospital Association, 1973), reprinted as B.C. Payne et al., *The Quality of Medical Care: Evaluation and Development* (Chicago: Hospital Research and Educational Trust, 1976).

13. R.H. Brook, *Quality of Care Assessment: A Comparison of Five Methods of Peer Review*, DHEW Publication No. HRA–74–1300 (Washington, D.C., U.S. Department of Health, Education, and Welfare, July, 1973).

14. R.H. Brook, "Effectiveness of Patient Care in an Emergency Room," *New England Journal of Medicine* 283, no. 17, (October 22, 1970): 904–907;

and R.H. Brook et al., "Effectiveness of Inpatient Follow-up Care," *New England Journal of Medicine* 285, no. 27 (December 30, 1971): 1509–14.

15. Robert H. Brook, "Critical Issues in the Assessment of Quality of Care," in Robert L. Kane, ed., *The Challenge of Community Medicine* (New York: Springer Publishing Co., Inc., 1974), pp. 183–211.

16. W.J. Fessel and E.E. Van Brunt, "Assessing Quality of Care from the Medical Record," *New England Journal of Medicine* 286, no. 3 (January 20, 1972): 134–38.

17. Martin S. Feldstein, *The Rising Cost of Hospital Care*, National Center for Health Services Research and Development, U.S. Dept. of Health, Education, and Welfare (Washington, D.C.: Information Resources Press, 1971).

18. A. Scitovsky and N. McCall, *Changes in the Costs of Treatments of Selected Illnesses*, NCHSR Research Digest Series, DHEW Publication No. HRA–77–3161 (Washington, D.C., U.S. Department of Health, Education, and Welfare, July 1976).

19. Ibid., p. 6.

20. Fessel and Van Brunt.

21. "Mortality Decline Increasing," *The Nation's Health*, May 1977, p. 7.

22. Final Mortality Statistics, 1976. Monthly Vital Statistics Report, Advance Report, National Center for Health Statistics, DHEW Publication No. (PHS) 78–1120, Vol. 26, No. 12, Supplement (2), March 30, 1978.

23. Victor R. Fuchs, *Who Shall Live?*

24. F. Cullen et al., "Survival and Follow-up Results in Critically Ill Patients," *New England Journal of Medicine* 294, no. 18 (April 29, 1976): 982–987.

25. Ibid., p. 982.

26. "Hospital Cost Fight Heats Up," *American Medical News*, June 2, 1978, p. 1.

27. *Length of Stay in PAS Hospitals, United States, 1972* (Ann Arbor: Commission on Professional and Hospital Activities, October 1973), p. 2.

28. Herbert E. Klarman, "Analysis of the HMO Proposal: Its Assumptions, Implications, and Prospects," in *Health Maintenance Organizations: A Reconfiguration of the Health Services System*, Proceedings of the Thirteenth Annual Symposium on Hospital Affairs, Center for Health Administration Studies University of Chicago, May 1971), pp. 24–38.

29. Harold S. Luft, *Trends in Medical Care Costs: Do HMO's Lower the Rate of Growth?* Department of Community and Preventive Medicine, Stanford University School of Medicine, Research Paper Series #77–6, October 1977. Stanford, CA.

30. R. Gibson and M. Mueller, "National Health Expenditures, Fiscal Year 1976," *Social Security Bulletin*, April 1977, pp. 3–22.

31. *Medical Care Expenditure: Prices and Costs, Background Book* (Washington, D.C.: DHEW, ORS/SSA, 1975).

32. Sherry Ellison-Cooke and Helen Thornberry, "Factors Affecting Nursing Home Medical Review: Implications for Program and Facility Planning," *Medical Care*, June 1977, pp. 494–504.

33. Thomas M. Tierney, Personal Communication, July 1978.

34. C.R. Gaus and F.J. Hellinger, "Results of Prospective Reimbursement," in W.L. Dowling, ed., *Topics in Health Care Financing*, Winter 1976. Vol. 3, No. 2: 83–96, Rockville, Md., Aspen Systems Corp.

35. R. Berry, "Prospective Rate Reimbursement and Cost Containment: Formula Reimbursement in New York," *Inquiry*, September 1976: 288–301.

36. A.P. Leco, *"Prospective Rate Setting in Rhode Island,"* in W.L. Dowling, ed., *Topics in Health Care Financing*, Winter 1976, pp. 39–56.

37. This section draws heavily on an analysis written by Jeanne Black.

38. C.C. Havinghurst, "Regulation of Health Facilities by Certificate of Need," *Virginia Law Review* 59 (1973): 1143–1232; C.C. Havinghurst, "Regulation of the Health Care System," *Hospitals, J.A.H.A.* 48 (1974): 65–71; W.J. Curran, *National Survey and Analysis of Certificate-of-Need Laws: Health Planning and Regulation in State Legislature 1972* (Chicago: American Hospital Association, Special Legislative Report, 1973); H.S. Cohen, "Regulating Health Care Facilities: the Certificate of Need Process Re-examined," *Inquiry* 10 (1973): 3–9; and A.E. Reider; J.R. Mason; and L.H. Glantz, "Certificate of Need: the Massachusetts Experience," *American Journal of Law and Medicine* 1 (March 1975): 13–40.

39. A complete summary and description of existing CON laws and regulation appears in W.J. Curran, "A National Survey and Analysis of State Certificate-of-Need Laws for Health Facilities," in C.C. Havinghurst, ed., *Regulating Health Facilities Construction* (Washington, D.C.: American Enterprise Institute for Public Policy Research, 1974), pp. 85–111.

40. United States Statutes At Large, Public Law 93–641, Section 1523, Paragraph (4), Washington, D.C., January 4, 1975.

41. F.J. Hellinger, "Effect of Certificate-of-Need Legislation on Hospital Investment," *Inquiry*, June 1976, pp. 187–93.

42. D.S. Salkever, and T.W. Bice, "Impact of State Certificate of Need Laws on Health Care Costs and Utilization" (Presented at the Eastern Economic Association meetings, Bloomsburg, Pennsylvania, April 17, 1976).

43. W.J. Bicknell, and D.C. Walsh, "Certificate-of-Need: The Massachusetts Experience," *New England Journal of Medicine*, May 15, 1975, pp. 1054–61.

44. Ibid., p. 1060.

45. Ibid.

46. *Expenditures for Health Care: Federal Programs and Their Effects* (Washington, D.C.: Congressional Budget Office, 1977).

47. G. Steuhler, "Certification of Need—A Systems Analysis of Maryland's Experience and Plans," *American Journal of Public Health*, November 1973, pp. 966–72.

48. Ibid., p. 971.

49. J.T. O'Connor, "Comprehensive Health Planning: Dreams and Realities," *Milbank Memorial Fund Quarterly*, Fall 1974.

50. Bicknell and Walsh, p. 1060.

51. C. Roseman, "Problems and Prospects of Comprehensive Health Planning," *American Journal of Public Health*, January 1972, pp. 16–19.

52. D.F. Phillips and K. Lille, "Putting the Leash on CAT: A Special Report," *Hospitals, J.A.H.A.* July 1, 1976, pp. 45–49. The interested reader will find this to be an excellent summary article on the current status of CT.

53. Ibid., p. 45.

54. G. Wartzman; R.C. Halgate; and P.P. Morgan, "Cranial Computed Tomography: An Evaluation of Cost Effectiveness," *Radiology*, October 1975, p. 75.

55. Ibid.

56. Herbert L. Abrams and Barbara J. McNeil, "Medical Implications of Computed Tomography," Parts I and II, *The New England Journal of Medicine* 298, nos. 5 and 6 (February 2 and 9, 1978).

57. Phillips and Lille., p. 48.

58. Institute of Medicine, "Assessing Quality in Health Care: an Evaluation" (Washington, D.C.: National Academy of Sciences, November 1976).

59. P. Gertman, Personal Communication, June 1977.

60. M. Bluestone and D.K. Baugh, "An Evaluation of a Medicare Concurrent Utilization Review Project: the Sacramento Certified Hospital Admission Program" (Baltimore: Office of Research and Statistics, Social Security Administration, 1977).

61. R.H. Brook and K.N. Williams, "Evaluation of the New Mexico Peer Review System, 1971 to 1973" (Santa Monica, CA.: Rand Corporation R−2110−HEW/RC, February 1977).

62. E.G. McCarthy, M.L. Finkel and A.S. Kamons, "Second Opinion Surgical Program: a Vehicle for Cost Containment?" Report of the National Commission on the Cost of Medical Care, Vol. II. Chicago, American Medical Association, 1978.

63. G. Janko, Bay State Health Care Foundation Inc., Personal Communication, June 1977.

64. McCarthy, Finkel and Kamons.

65. Ibid.

66. P.B. Ginsburg, "Impact of the Economic Stabilization Program on Hospitals: An Analysis with Aggregate Data," in *Hospital Cost Containment: Selected Notes for Future Policy*, M. Zubkoff, I.E. Raskin, and R.S. Hanft, eds. (New York: PRODIST (published for the Milbank Memorial Fund in cooperation with the National Center for Health Services Research), 1978.

67. R.G. Evans, "Beyond the Medical Market Place: Expenditure, Utilization, and Pricing of Insured Health Care in Canada," in R.N. Rosett, *The Role of Health Insurance in the Health Services Sector* (New York: National Bureau of Economic Research, 1976), pp. 437−93.

68. Ibid., p. 465.

69. *Hospital Statistics: Annual Preliminary Report* (Canada: Dominion Bureau of Statistics, Department of National Health and Welfare, #83−217, 1975 and 1976).

Chapter 4

1. *Congressional Record—House*, April 25, 1977, p. H−3527, Summary of HR 6575.

2. Ibid., p. H−3528.

3. Ibid., p. H−3531.

4. Ibid., p. H−3528.

5. Ibid.

6. Ibid., p. H−3529.

7. Ibid.

8. Ibid., p. H−3527.

9. For example, revenues in 1978 are permitted to increase by 9 percent of 1976's revenue per admission, which is equivalent to a 7.83 percent increase over 1977 revenue because 1977 revenue is 115 percent of 1976 revenue, i.e., 9.00 = 7.83 × 115.

10. M. Feldstein, "Quality of Hospital Services: An Analysis of Geographic Variation and Intertemporal Change," in M. Perlman, ed., *The Economy of Health and Medical Care* (London: MacMillan, 1974).

11. American Hospital Association, "Guide to the AHA's Program for Monitoring the Hospital Economy" (Chicago: 1974); and later unpublished tables.

12. Victor R. Fuchs, "The Earnings of Allied Health Personnel: Are Health Workers Underpaid?" *Explorations in Economic Research* 3, no. 3 (Summer 1976): 408−32.

13. D.E. Yett, "The Chronic 'Shortage' of Nurses: A Public Policy Dilemma," in H.E. Klarman, ed., *Empirical Studies in Health Economics: Proceedings of the Second Conference on the Economics of Health* (Baltimore: Johns Hopkins Press, 1970).

14. Martin S. Feldstein, *The Rising Cost of Hospital Care*, National Center for Health Services Research and Development, U.S. Department of Health, Education, and Welfare (Washington, D.C.: Information Resources Press, 1971).

15. P. Feldstein, "An Empirical Investigation of the Marginal Cost of Hospital Services" (Chicago: Graduate Program in Hospital Administration, University of Chicago, 1961).

16. J.R. Lave, and L.B. Lave, "Hospital Cost Functions," *American Economic Review*, June 1970, pp. 379−95; M. Ingbar and L. Taylor, *Hospital Costs in Massachusetts* (Cambridge, Massachusetts: Harvard University Press, 1968); and M. Feldstein, *Economic Analysis for Health Services Efficiency* (Amsterdam: North Holland Publishing Company, 1967).

17. R.F. Conrad, "Modeling the Short-Run Behavior of the Hospital Industry Using a Joint Cost Function" (Madison: University of Wisconsin, February 1977).

18. In a subsequent version of the administration's proposal, this limit was changed to a simple 2 to 1 ratio of current assets to liabilities.

19. *Congressional Record—House*, April 25, 1977, p. H−3529, Summary of HR 6575.

Chapter 5

1. S. 1470, A Bill in the Senate of the United States, May 5, 1977, p. 4.

2. Ibid.

3. Ibid.

4. Ibid., p. 6.

5. Ibid., p. 3.

6. Ibid., p. 5−6.

7. Ibid., p. 7.

8. Ibid., p. 8.

9. For a further discussion of how a comprehensive efficiency adjustment could be incorporated into the administration's proposal, see Appendix B.

10. S 1470, p. 10–11.

11. Ibid., p. 10.

Chapter 6

1. J.D. Thompson; C.D. Mross; and R.B. Fetter, "Case Mix and Resource Use" (New Haven: Center for the Study of Health Services, Yale University Institution for Social and Policy Studies, 1975).

2. For a description of the various approaches, see K.R. Kosnik, "Methodology and Empirical Validation of a Multidimensional Hospital Classification Structure" (Ph.D. Dissertation, Northwestern University, 1975), pp. 84–88.

3. President's Hospital Cost Containment Proposal (HR 6575): Joint Hearings Before the Subcommittee on Health, Committee on Ways and Means and the Subcommittee on Health and the Environment, Committee on Interstate and Foreign Commerce, U.S. House of Representatives, 95th Cong., May 11, 12, and 13, 1977, p. 669.

Appendix B

1. This assumes that the formula originally included in the administration proposal is replaced by a limit that is the sum of the increase in the GNP deflator plus an explicitly allowed increase in intensity and expansion of service equal to the real growth of GNP (that is, 3 percent); see page 79 for a criticism of the original administration formula for calculating the national revenue limit.

2. *Selected Hospital Cost Containment Proposals: Major Provisions* (Washington, D.C.: Committee on Finance, U.S. Senate, October 11, 1977), p. 1.

3. P.J. Phillip and R.N. Iyer, "Classification of Community Hospitals," *Health Services Research* 10, no. 4 (Winter 1975): 349–68.

Index

About the Authors

Edward F.X. Hughes, Director of the Center for Health Services and Policy Research, is a physician. He is Clinical Professor of Community Medicine in Northwestern's Medical School, and Professor of Hospital and Health Services Management in the Graduate School of Management's Program in Hospital and Health Services Management.

David P. Baron is an economist and decision theorist, and is Professor of Managerial Economics and Decision Sciences in the Graduate School of Management.

David A. Dittman is an accountant and is now Associate Professor in the Graduate School of Business Administration, Duke University.

Bernard S. Friedman is an economist and Assistant Professor of Economics.

Beaufort B. Longest, Jr. is an organizational theorist and specialist in hospital administration. He is Associate Professor of Hospital and Health Services Management in the Program in Hospital and Health Services Management.

Mark V. Pauly is an economist and Professor of Economics.

Kenneth R. Smith is the Director of the Program in Hospital and Health Services Management and Professor of Managerial Economics and Decision Sciences in the Graduate School of Management.